PHYSICAL WISDOM

Kundalini Yoga as Taught by Yogi Bhajan®

Compiled and Illustrated by: Harijot Kaur Khalsa

Managing Editor: Ardas Kaur Khalsa

KRI Reviewer: Gurucharan Singh Khalsa

Senior Editors: Gurucharan Singh Khalsa
Shakti Parwha Kaur Khalsa
Pritpal Kaur Khalsa

Book Design and Production: Khalsa Marketing Group

Yogi Bhajan Photo: Satsimran Kaur

Published by **Kundalini Research Institute**, PO Box 1819, Santa Cruz, NM 87567

ISBN 978-1-934532-03-4

Acknowledgements

The technology of Kundalini Yoga and White Tantric Yoga was brought to the West from India by the grace of Siri Singh Sahib Bhai Sahib Harbhajan Singh Khalsa Yogiji (Yogi Bhajan). The teachings in this manual are entirely his gift. We wish to gratefully acknowledge his gift and the inspiration he offered to us all in manifesting our highest potential. Any errors or omissions in this manual are entirely the fault of the Editors and by no means reflect upon the perfection and comprehensiveness of the teachings.

The yoga sets in this manual are classes taught by Yogi Bhajan and are available on audio, DVD and VHS. Although every effort has been made to communicate the technology of these classes accurately, nothing replaces the experience of doing Kundalini Yoga with the Master, Yogi Bhajan. We suggest that you enhance your yoga experience by collecting DVDs of one or more of your favorite sets from this manual. There is something about doing Kundalini Yoga in the presence of the Master, Yogi Bhajan (even on video) that brings out the best yogi within you. Contact Ancient Healing Ways, Store.a-healing.com for information about purchasing DVDs or audio cassettes or see www.kriteachings.org.

KRI Seal of Approval

Kundalini Research Institute

"This Seal of Approval is granted only to those products which have been approved through the KRI review process for accuracy and integrity of those portions which embody the technology of Kundalini Yoga and 3HO Lifestyle as taught by Yogi Bhajan."

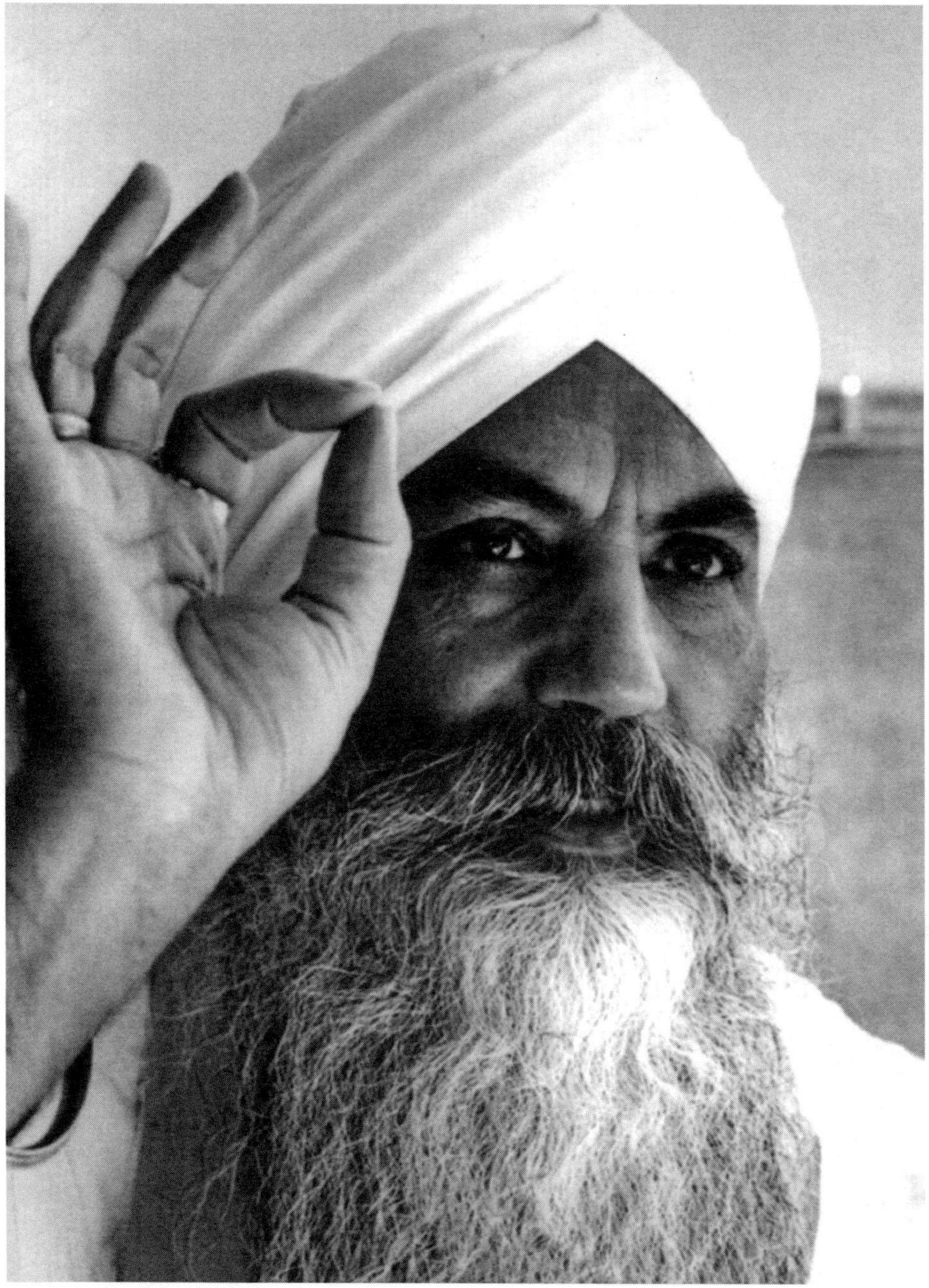

Physical Wisdom

Body Affects the Soul.
Soul Affects the Mind.

Creative action is like this:
we can grow either through the meditative way
or the physical way.
The meditative way will be very polite.
It takes a long time
and it needs a lot of discipline and endurance.
The physical way is here and now,
immediate and effective.
Which way do you choose?

INTRODUCTION

For Beginners

If you are a beginning student of Kundalini Yoga, practicing for less than six months, or if you have been practicing without the aid of a KRI certified teacher, please read this introduction before you begin to practice from this instruction manual.

Sadhana Guidelines

This manual has been prepared as a supplement and extension to Kundalini Yoga Sadhana Guidelines, 2nd Edition, in which Yogi Bhajan explains yoga, meditation, and the energy that is Kundalini. Also important for beginners are the descriptions of the basics of Kundalini Yoga: asanas (postures), mudras (hand positions), bandhas (energy locks), and mantras (sound currents) written by Gurucharan Singh Khalsa, Director of Training for the Kundalini Research Institute's Aquarian Trainer Academy.

The Teacher

Kundalini Yoga is a spiritual discipline which cannot be practiced without a teacher. However it is not necessary for the teacher to be physically present when you practice. To establish a creative link with the Master of Kundalini Yoga, Yogi Bhajan, you should be sure to tune in to his energy flow using the Adi Mantra, *Ong Namo Guru Dev Namo.*

Tuning In

Every Kundalini Yoga session begins with chanting the Adi Mantra: *Ong Namo Guru Dev Namo.* By chanting it in its proper form and consciousness, the student becomes open to the higher Self, the source of all guidance, and accesses the protective link between himself or herself and the divine teacher.

How to Recite the Adi Mantra

Sit in a comfortable cross-legged position with the spine straight. Place the palms of the hands together as if in prayer, with the fingers pointing straight up, and then press the joints of the thumbs into the center of the chest, at the sternum. Inhale deeply. Focus your concentration at the root of the nose between the eyebrows, your Brow Point. As you exhale, chant the entire mantra in one breath. If your breath is not capable of this, take a quick sip of air through the mouth after "Ong Namo" and then chant the rest of the mantra, extending the sound as long as possible. The sound "Dev" is chanted a minor third higher than the other sounds of the mantra.

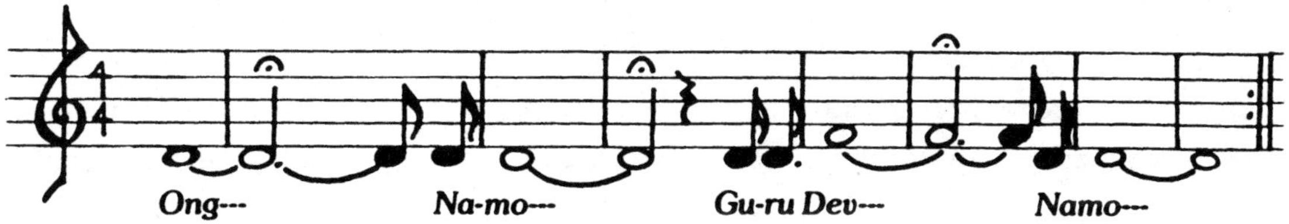

As you chant, vibrate the cranium with the sound to create a mild pressure at the Brow Point or third eye. Chant this mantra at least three times before beginning your Kundalini Yoga practice. See www.kriteachings.org to hear a sample of the Director of Training leading the Adi Mantra.

Pronunciation

The "O" sound in *Ong* is long, as in "go" and of short duration. The "ng" sound is long and produces a definite vibration on the roof of the mouth and cranium. The first part of *Namo*, is short and rhymes with "hum." The "O", as in "go" is held longer.
The first syllable of *Guru* is pronounced as in the word, "good." The second syllable rhymes with "true." The first syllable is short and the second one long. The word, *Dev*, rhymes with "gave."

Definition

Ong is the infinite creative energy experienced in manifestation and activity. It is a variation of the cosmic syllable *Om* which denotes God in an absolute or unmanifested state. God as Creator is called *Ong.*

Namo has the same root as the Sanskrit word *Namaste* which means reverent greetings.

Namaste is a common greeting in India accompanied by the palms pressed together at the chest or forehead. It implies bowing down. Together *Ong Namo* means "I call on the infinite creative consciousness," and opens you to the universal consciousness that guides all action.

Guru is the embodiment of the wisdom that one is seeking. The Guru is the giver of the technology. *Dev* means higher, subtle, or divine. It refers to the transparent or spiritual realms.

Namo, in closing the mantra, reaffirms the humble reverence of the student. Taken together, *Guru Dev Namo* means "I call on the divine wisdom," whereby you bow before your higher Self to guide you in using the knowledge and energy given by the cosmic Self.

Mental Focus

The following pages contain many wonderful techniques. To fully appreciate and receive the benefits of each one you will need mental focus. Unless you are directed to do otherwise, focus your concentration on the Brow Point, which is located between the eyebrows just above the root of the nose. With your eyes closed, mentally locate this point by turning your eyes gently upwards and inwards. Remain aware of your breath, your body posture, your movements, and any mantra you may be using, even as you center your awareness at the Brow Point or third eye.

Linking the Breath With a Mantra

A mantra is a sequence of sounds designed to direct the mind by their rhythmic repetition. To fully utilize the power of mantra, link the mantra with your breath cycle. A basic mantra is Sat Nam (rhymes with "But Mom"). *Sat Nam* means "Truth is my identity." Mentally repeat "Sat" as you inhale, and "Nam" as you exhale. In this way you filter your thoughts so that each thought has a positive resolution. Mantra makes it easier to keep up during strenuous exercises and adds depth to the performance of even the simplest ones.

Pacing Yourself

Kundalini Yoga often involves the rhythmic movement between two or more postures. Begin slowly, keeping a steady rhythm. Increase gradually, being careful not to strain. Usually the more you practice an exercise, the faster you can go. Just be sure that the spine has become warm and flexible before attempting rapid movements. It is important to be aware of your body and to be responsible for its well-being.

Concluding an Exercise

Unless otherwise stated, an exercise is concluded by inhaling and holding the breath briefly, then exhaling and relaxing the posture. While the breath is being held, apply the Mulbandh or Root Lock, contracting the muscles around the anus, the sex organs, and the Navel Point. This consolidates the effects of any exercise and circulates the energy to your higher centers. Do not hold the breath to the point of dizziness. If you start to feel dizzy or faint, immediately exhale and relax.

Relaxation Between Exercises

An important part of any exercise is the relaxation following it. Unless otherwise specified, you should allow 1 to 3 Minutes of relaxation in Easy Pose or lying on the back in Corpse Pose after each exercise. The less experienced you are or the more strenuous the exercise, the longer the relaxation period should be. Some sets end with a period of "deep relaxation" which may extend from 3 to 10 Minutes.

Music

See Appendix A for information on where to get music played in various sets. If you do not have the specific tape played in a set you may substitute other meditative music or do the set without music.

On Your Way...

The exercises in this manual are designed to be safe for most people, provided the instructions are followed carefully. The benefits attributed to these exercises come from centuries-old yogic tradition. Results will vary due to physical differences and the correctness and frequency of practice. The publishers and authors disclaim all liability in connection with the use of the information in individual cases. As with all unsupervised exercise programs, your use of the instructions in this manual is taken at your own risk. If you have any doubts as to the suitability of the exercises, please consult a doctor.

We invite you to now enjoy the practice of the Kundalini Yoga techniques contained in the following pages. If you have any questions or concerns about your practice of Kundalini Yoga, please contact your local KRI Certified teacher.

Table of Contents

Foreword

by Harijot Kaur Khalsa

The ancient yogis and sages who developed Kundalini Yoga had a deep respect for the Creator of this human body. They knew, in their profound devotion and worship, that so perfect a Creator could only have created perfection in design, function and potential. Based on this respect, they sought knowledge of the totality of the human being. They researched the human ability to maintain good health, increase vitality, open consciousness and expand the experience of the excellence of human life. Their research gave them a great understanding of the nervous system, glandular system, organ system, energy system and the brain. They learned how blood, nerves, muscles, organs, and glands all work together. They investigated the seen and the unseen, and the interrelationships between the physical and the subtle. From this research they developed Kundalini Yoga.

Kundalini Yoga is a highly evolved technology based on a thorough understanding of the ecology of the human body, how the breath affects the thinking, how the angle of a finger affects the pituitary gland, and so on. This technology works with the systems of the human body using the body's own means. Hand position, breath, posture, sound, and motion are employed in various ways to create the optimum balance among all the body's components. Kundalini Yoga gives us access to the full resources of this perfectly designed human body and deepens our appreciation of this body as a miraculous gift.

The techniques of Kundalini Yoga were discovered and practiced through many ages by thousands of sages, saints, and healers. Until recent times these techniques had been secret, taught only to a chosen few. Yogi Bhajan believed that these techniques of physical wisdom belong to us all and that access to this wisdom is our birthright as human beings. In the following collection of yoga sets and meditations, you will experience a small portion of this timeless physical wisdom that is the legacy of the teachings of Yogi Bhajan.

We are accustomed to wisdom that is expressed in words. Kundalini Yoga is wisdom expressed through the medium of action. It can only speak to you if you do it. This ancient and priceless wisdom will give you the experience of the unfolding of your own inner wisdom as you use your physical body in the practice of Kundalini Yoga.

Self-Healing

December 11, 1985

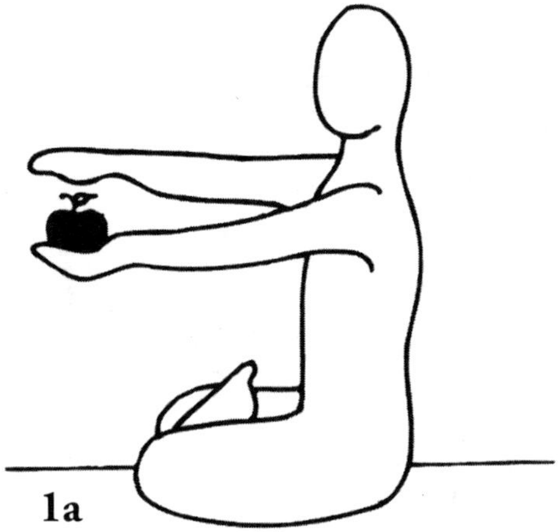

1a

You'll need either an apple or a banana for this set.

1. Sit in Easy Pose with your arms stretched straight out in front. Put your fruit in your right hand (if you are male) or your left hand (if you are female). With the opposite hand cover the fruit, keeping your hand about 4 to 6 inches above it. Keep your arms straight with no bend in the elbows. Close your eyes, go inward, and concentrate. Create a connection between the navel and the fruit so that you gather the energy of the navel and project it in blessing into the fruit. This is for self-healing. The *praan*, the life force energy, lives in the Navel Point. You are taking that life force and blessing the fruit. With the hand above, you bless the fruit below. There will be a lot of obstructions in doing this: body won't participate, mind won't concentrate, and you won't like it. Between the three, bring out a balance.

Fruit is often used as a kind of psychic storage device. Fruit is etheric and grows well above the earth. It has a subtle quality that lets it easily absorb pranic energy and become a useful tool in healing exercises.

Gurucharan Singh

To add strength to yourself (it is not absolutely necessary), play Ragi Sat Nam Singh's *Jaap Sahib.* 9 Minutes.

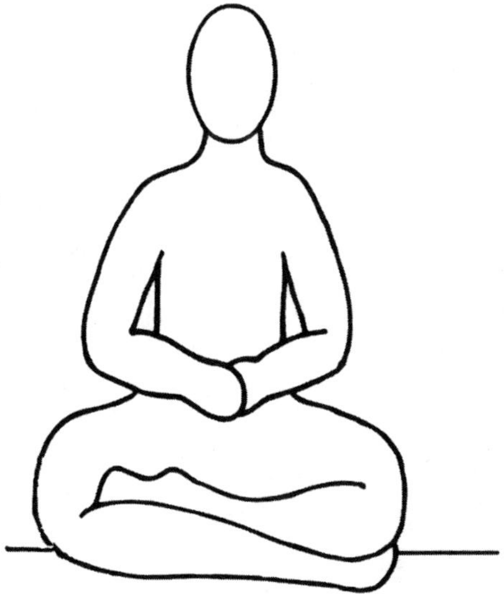

1b

2. Hold your fruit between both hands and place it at your Navel Point. Breathe as long and as deeply as you can in this position for 2 Minutes. With the fruit still at your navel, inhale as deeply as you can, hold the breath as long as you can, exhale long and deep, and hold your breath out as long as you can. Give a conscious rhythm to your breath. 7 Minutes.

To finish: Inhale, press your fruit against your navel (If you have a banana, be careful not to squash it) and press your tongue hard against your upper palate. Exhale and eat your fruit. To maximize the self-healing benefits of this set, do it for 90 days as your breakfast. Eat only this fruit and a cup or glass of yogi tea with a moderate amount of milk but no honey. Then do not eat anything else until noon.

Self-Renewal

May 17, 1992

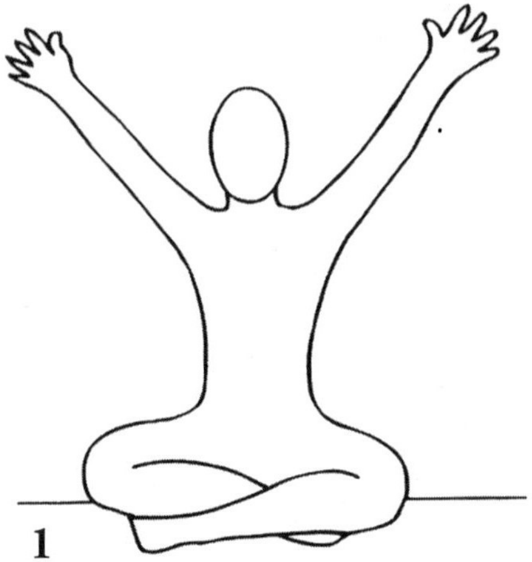

1

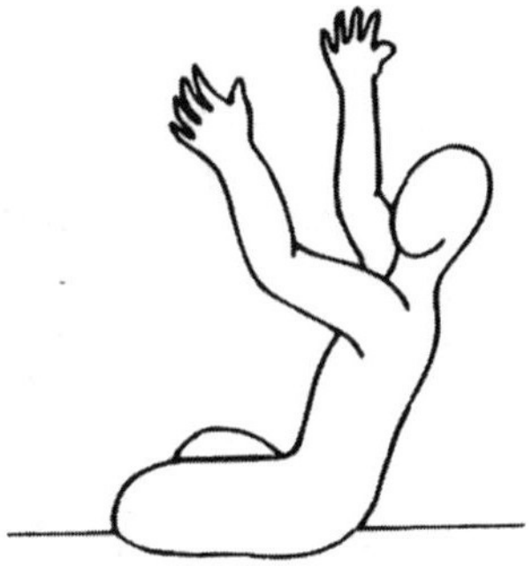

Side view of Exercise 1

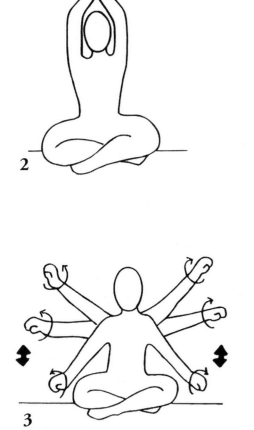

2

3

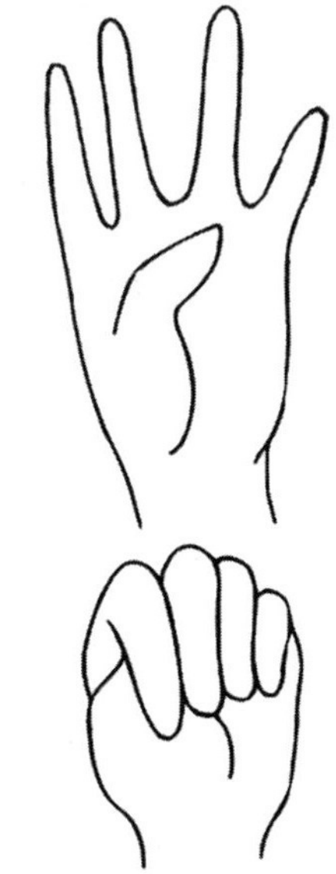

Mudra for Exercise 3

1. To balance the sugar and sodium in your body: Sit in Easy Pose and lean backward. Your head is slightly back, your chin is in and your chest is out. There will be a pressure in the shoulder blade area. Spread your arms wide, with the fingers open. Be relaxed and full of ecstasy with no stiffness in your muscles. Begin Breath of Fire from your Navel Point, really move the navel with each breath. After 3 Minutes, open your mouth and stick out your tongue and continue Breath of Fire for another 2 Minutes.

2. To stretch the spine and keep you youthful and healthy: Sit in Easy Pose with the arms stretched over your head with the palms touching. Stretch, pulling the spine, rib cage, and armpits upward. Fight gravity with your own will and keep stretching up for 3 Minutes. Don't let the palms separate. (This exercise may be increased up to a total of 5 Minutes, but no longer unless you have a full hour to relax afterward.)

3. To balance the glandular system (must be done in conjunction with exercises 1 & 2): Touch your thumbs to the mound below your Sun finger (ring finger) and close your other fingers around them to form a fist. Lean back as in Exercise 1. Stretch your arms out to the sides and begin quickly revolving your arms backward in small circles, keeping your elbows straight but not locked. Continue to make the backward circles as you raise and lower both arms at the same time. There should be pressure between your shoulder blades. 7 Minutes.

Is yoga a religion? It is and it is not. In religion you have to believe something and in yoga you have to experience what you want to believe.

Yogi Bhajan

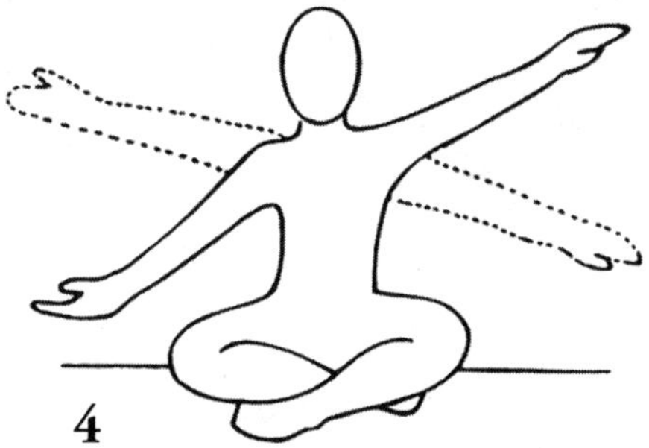

4

4. To loosen up your spine and to balance the left and right hemispheres of your brain: Sitting in Easy Pose, stretch your arms straight out to the sides so that your arms are in one straight line. Turn your left palm down and your right palm up. Keeping the arms in one straight line, raise one arm as the other one is lowered (like a seesaw). Move as quickly as you can.
3 Minutes.

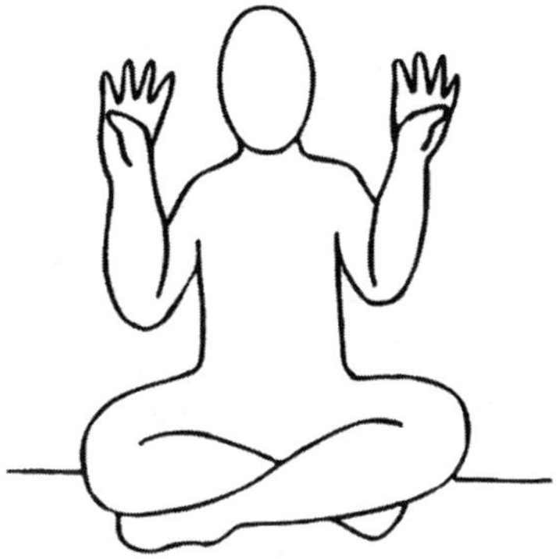

5

5. Sit in Easy Pose and bend your elbows so that your hands are up by your ears. Put the thumb on the mound below the Mercury finger (pinkie) and keep the fingers pointing straight up, the fingers are not touching each other. Close your eyes, look at your chin with your closed eyes, and pretend to watch one of your fantasies played on a screen in your chin. (You will never have a nightmare if this meditation is perfected.) Relax and meditate for 11 Minutes, listening to Nirinjan Kaur's "Chattr Chakkr Varti." Breathe long, slow, and deep. After 11 Minutes, inhale, hold your breath, and tighten every muscle of your body as you sit in the posture. Exhale and repeat this 2 more times.

6. Stand up and dance. Shake and loosen every part of your body for 3-5 Minutes to spread the benefits of the meditations all over your body.

7

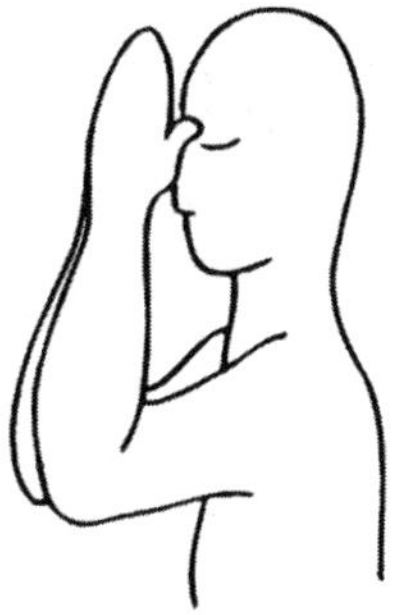

7. Sit in Easy Pose and put your hands in Prayer Pose. The thumbs are gently placed on the part of the eye socket where the eyebrow begins at the side of the bridge of the nose. Don't press too hard here. Chant *Ong Namo, Guru Dev Namo* [Nirinjan Kaur's version was used in class] for 3 Minutes. Inhale, hold your breath 10 seconds and exhale. Repeat this 2 more times.

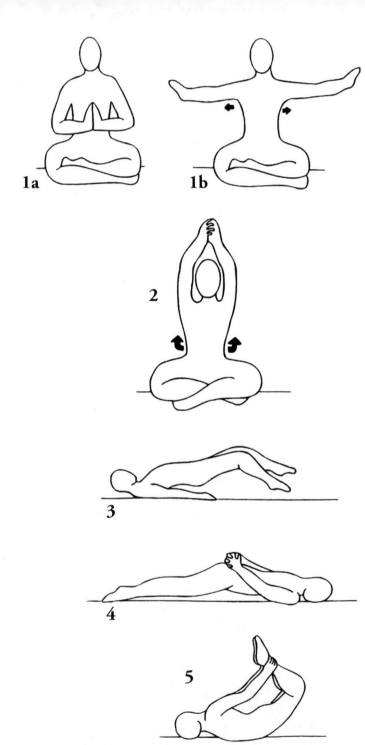

1a

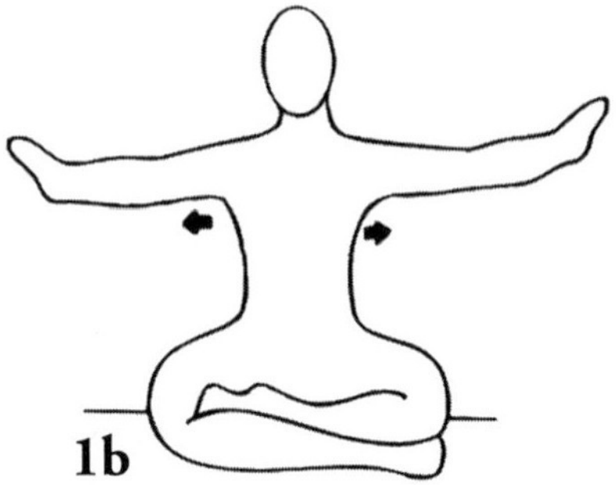

1b

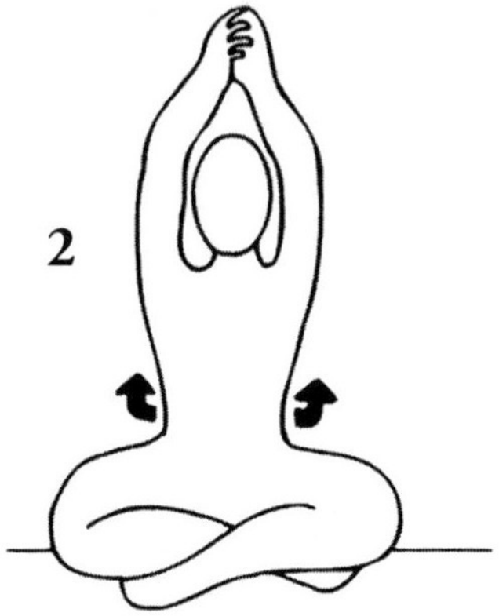

2

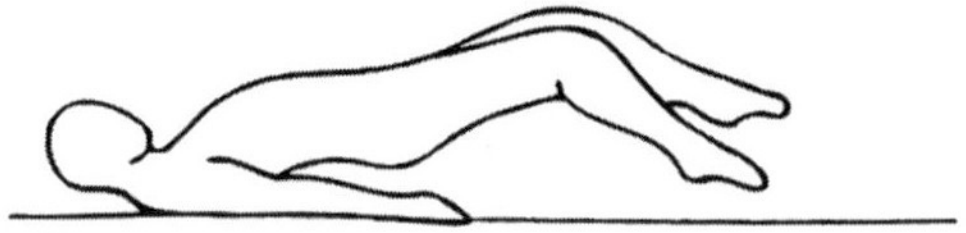

3

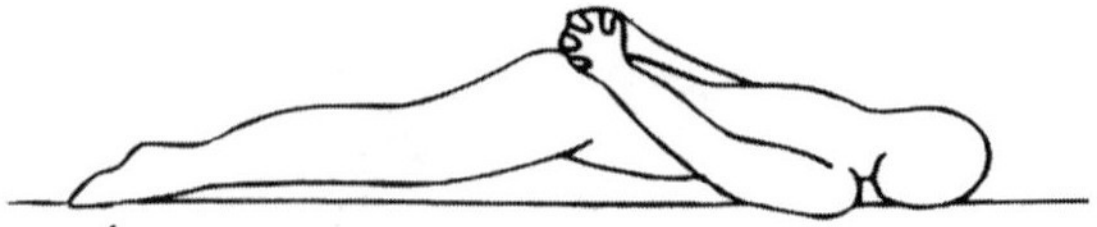

4

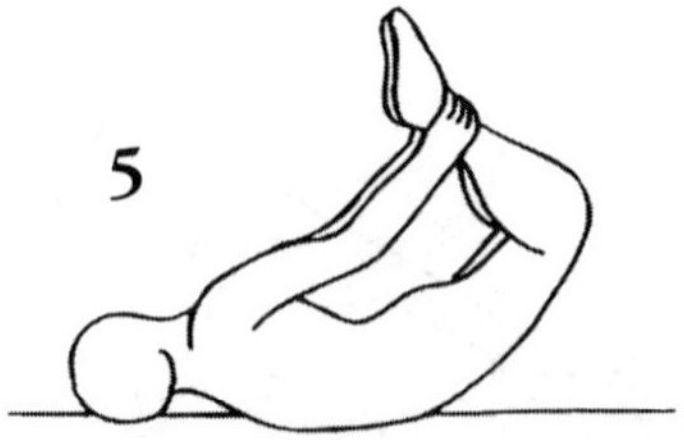

5

Strengthen the Immune System I

October 22, 1985

1. Sitting in Easy Pose, bring your hands into Prayer Pose at the center of your chest and then extend your arms out to the sides. Return them to Prayer Pose and continue, stretching the armpits as much as you can when you extend the arms out to the sides. Breathe long and deep. Keep moving faster and faster, extending the arms all the way out. You are exercising your immune system and making it stronger. After 3 Minutes, start getting angry and feisty. Start fighting and use the motion to get all your anger out. Continue for another 8 Minutes.

2. Sitting in Easy Pose, interlace your fingers to lock your hands above your head with your elbows straight. Twist left and right from the base of your spine. Do Breath of Fire and move wildly. 4 Minutes. This is very good for the liver.

3. Lie down on your back and make your body jump vigorously up, down, and all around. Move every part of your body including your head. Move vigorously. This is the best exercise to get rid of anger and it makes the immune system healthy. 4 Minutes.

4. Turn onto your belly and lock your hands in the small of your back. Again make your body jump vigorously up, down, and all around. Move every part of you. 3 1/2 Minutes.

5. Keeping your forehead on the floor, grab your ankles and pull up on them so that you lift your knees up from the ground. Once you are balanced with your knees suspended, hold the posture with a long, slow breath for 1 1/2 Minutes.

6. Turn over onto your back and nap, listening to "Naad - the Blessing" by Sangeet Kaur Khalsa. After 11 Minutes begin to sing along for another 4 Minutes. In class Yogi Bhajan played the gong during this meditation.

It is self-control which matters in life. Life is not given to you for any other reason but to experience your own creativity and your own Self in the dignity of its existence.

Yogi Bhajan

Strengthen the Immune System II

October 23, 1985

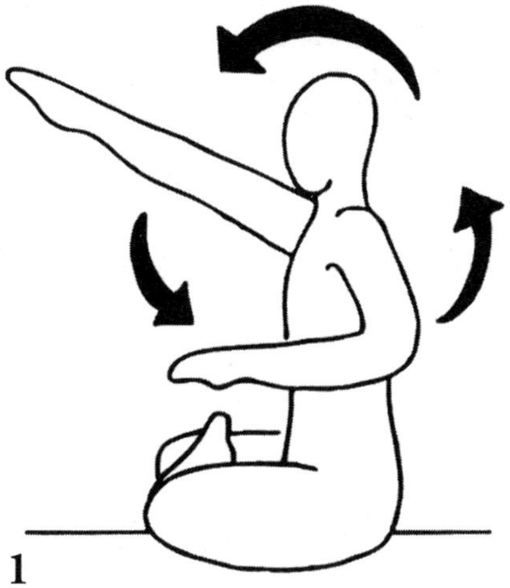

1

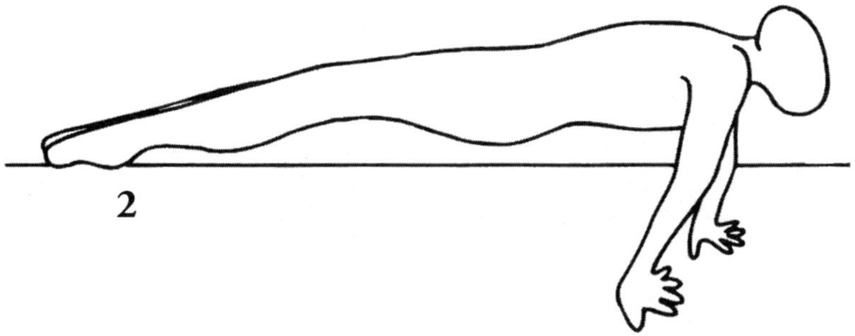

2

1. This special breath exercise is called "Swimming through the Pranic Ocean." Sit in Easy Pose and move the arms like you are swimming. Extend one and then the other in constant motion. As one arm extends, the other draws back with the elbow along your side. Do not punch. Create a smooth, circular swimming motion that moves the shoulders, rib cage, and back muscles. Create a powerful Breath of Fire through an open mouth in rhythm with the arm motion. Keep the back molars together so the breath sounds like a powerful, pulsing hiss. Continue for 13 Minutes.

2. Come into back platform pose. Keep your body straight, especially your knees. Let your neck relax backwards but do not let it hyper-extend or crimp. This puts pressure on the parathyroid. After 2 Minutes, form a circle with your mouth and breathe strongly. Puff in and out using the diaphragm to drive the breath. This is not a Breath of Fire from the navel, it is a "pancreas breath" that is focused near the sternum and diaphragm. Continue for another 2 Minutes.

3. Lie down straight and nap in Corpse Pose. 17 Minutes.

4. While still lying down, play Liv Singh's "Har Har Mukande" with affirmations and repeat the affirmations that Yogi Bhajan recites at the beginning. Then stretch, twist around, move your shoulders, and wake up dancing. 3 Minutes.

5. Come into a sitting position and dance while sitting. This spreads the energy equally to all parts of the body. 1 1/2 Minutes.

Your immune system works for you, but do you work for your immune system? Your heart works for you. Do you work for your heart? Your organs work for you. Do you work for each of your organs? I don't think you have asked yourself questions like these.

Yogi Bhajan

Change the Ions in the Body

May 21, 1986

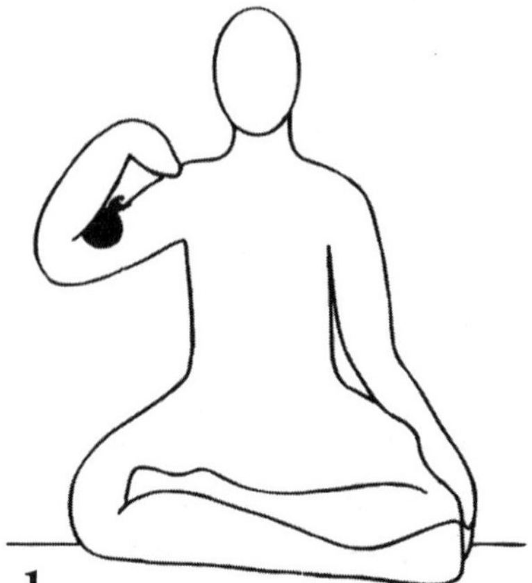
1

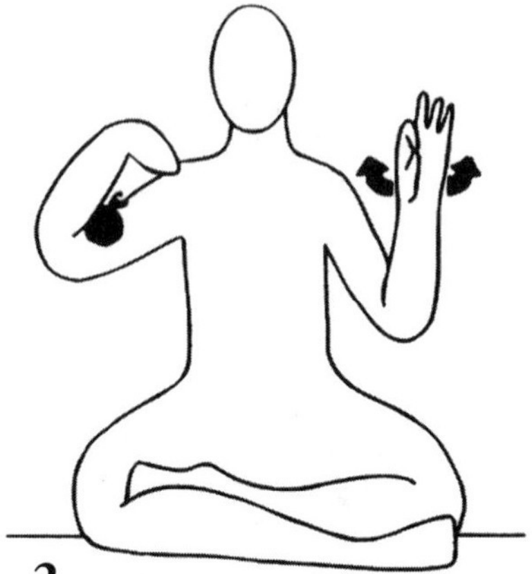
2

You will need a small to medium sized apple for this set.

1. Sit in Easy Pose. With your right arm out to the side, place your apple in the crook of your elbow and close your arm around it. You will press hard on the apple. The fingertips of the right hand touch your right shoulder. 2 Minutes.

2. Keeping your right arm in the same position, bend your left elbow and bring your left hand up a little above shoulder height. Put your left hand in Gyan Mudra and begin twisting this hand left and right at the wrist. Do Breath of Fire and move the hand quickly. 4 1/2 Minutes.

3. Staying in the same posture and continuing to rotate your left hand, begin twisting left and right from the base of your spine. Continue Breath of Fire. 5 1/2 Minutes.

4. Lie down flat. Put the apple on your navel and press it hard with both hands (one on top of the other). The apple should disappear into your belly. Pump your navel, keeping the downward pressure on the apple with your hands. 3 Minutes.

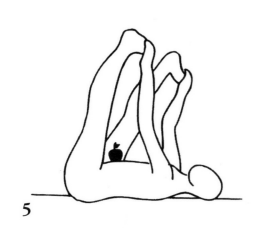

5

5. Leave the apple at your navel. Lift your legs and spread them wide. Grab onto your toes and balance on your spine. Tighten your belly and press your navel up against the apple. If the posture is correct the apple will sit, if it's wrong, the apple will slip. Go to sleep in this posture. 9 Minutes. Yogi Bhajan played the gong during this meditative nap.

6

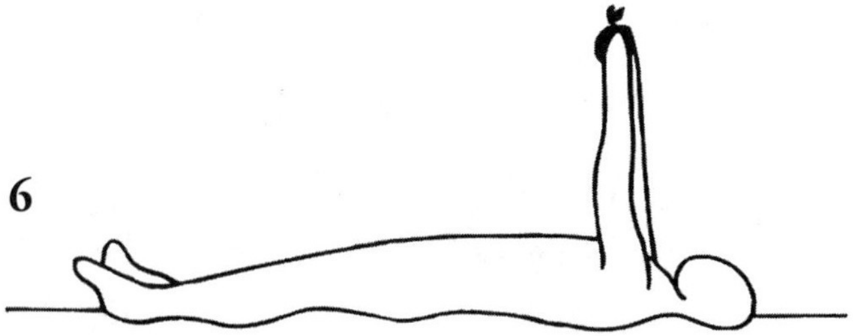

6. Lie flat and stretch your legs out straight. Take the apple in both hands and hold your arms straight up. Allow no bend in the elbows. Listen to "Walking Up the Mountain with You" by Gurudass Singh and Krishna Kaur. 7 1/2 Minutes.

7. Rise up and eat your apple. Chew it well. 3-5 Minutes.

Life is experienced in direct proportion to your mental love. If you love a great ideal, you become great. If you love a small thing, you become small.

Yogi Bhajan

The Healing Strength of the Inner Self

October 9, 1985

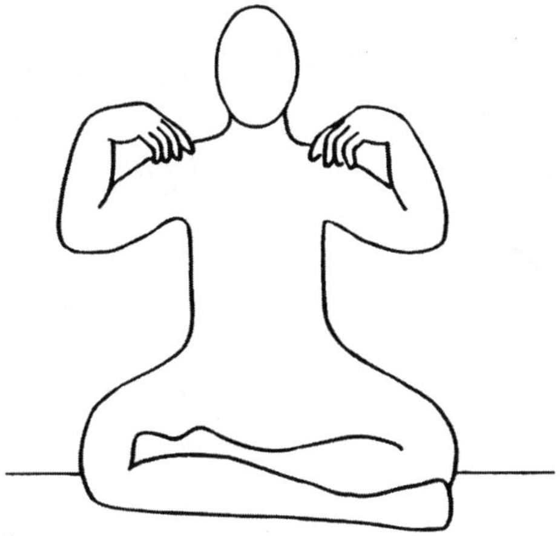

1

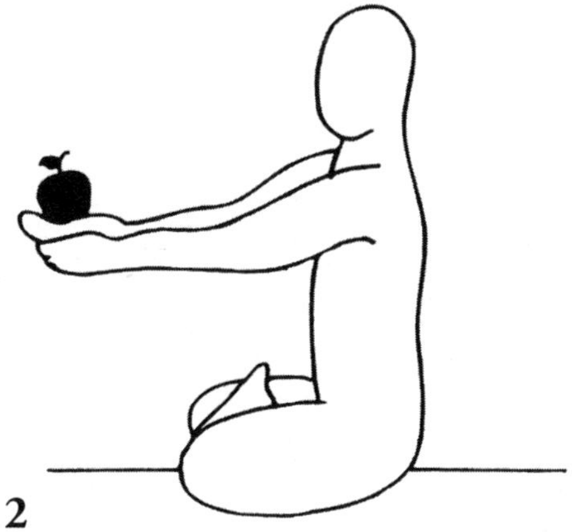

2

You will need a piece of fruit for this exercise. Apple, banana, pear, grapes, it is your choice.

1. Sit in Easy Pose with a straight spine and put your fingertips on your shoulders. Your elbows point to each side and are at shoulder level. Close your eyes and, breathing through the nose, inhale in eight strokes and exhale in eight strokes. Keep your spine straight. 5 1/2 Minutes.

2. Extend both arms straight out in front of you with the hands together palms facing up, the left hand is under the right. Your fruit is in the palm of the right hand. Keep your arms straight with no bend in the elbows. Close your eyes and concentrate. Inhale in eight strokes and exhale in eight strokes. 5 1/2 Minutes.

Inhale deeply, stretch your hands out, hold the breath for 10 seconds, and exhale. Eat your fruit. Sit and relax for 11 Minutes.

In these 22 Minutes you can effectively call on your inner reserve of energy to heal and elevate yourself. The deep physical wisdom and intelligence in your design is available to you if you call on it. The eight stroke breath invokes the creative link between the earth and the ether, between the subtle and the coarse aspects of one's self.

Gurucharan Singh

The caliber of this human body is such that it has the capacity to give you the experience of God.

Yogi Bhajan

Massage for the Lymphatic System

October 30, 1985

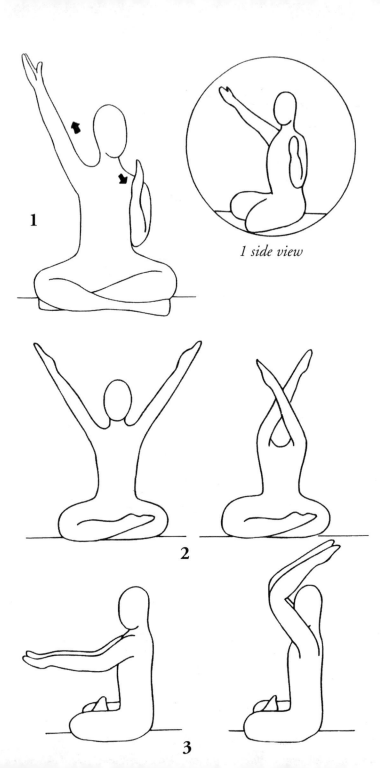

1

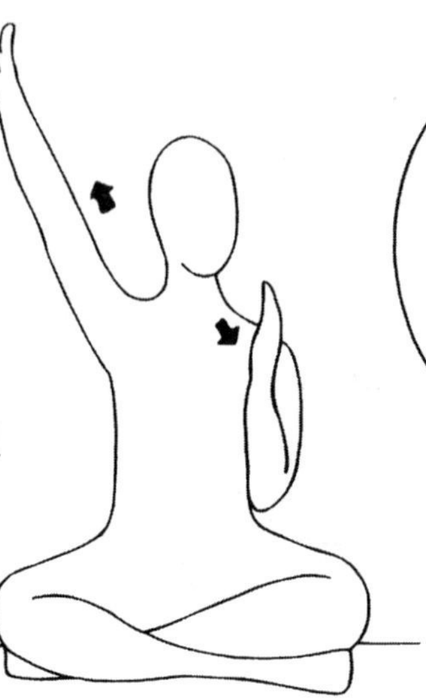

1 side view

2

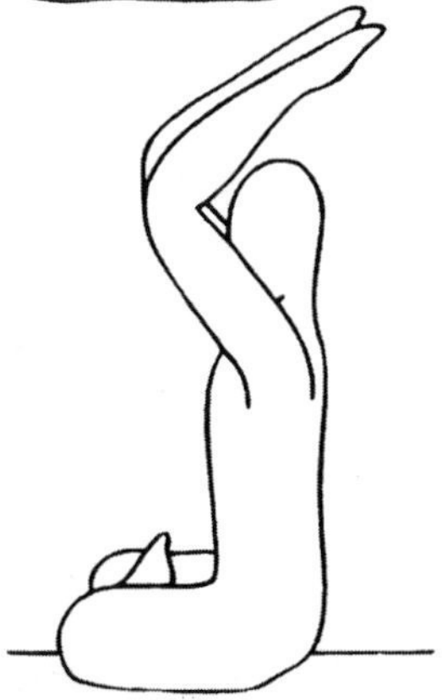

3

1. Sit in Easy Pose. Keeping the arms close to your sides, bend the elbows so that the hands and forearms are pointing straight up and the palms are facing each other. Strongly push one arm out and up at a 60 degree angle while the other arm remains bent, becomes hard like steel, and creates a solid balance for the extended arm. Then push out the bent arm while the extended arm returns to the balancing position close in to the side of the body. The arm is pushed out from the armpit, which is stretched in this motion. This is a very vigorous and demanding exercise. You will work hard to do it correctly. You are channelizing the energy of the *Ida* and *Pingala*. 10 Minutes.

2. Extend both arms up and out, creating a V between your arms. Keep the elbows straight and criss-cross your arms in front of your face. Move very quickly with Breath of Fire. 1 1/2 Minutes.

3. Extend both arms out in front of you with the palms facing up. Move both arms together, as if you were splashing water up and over your head. Breathe powerfully through your mouth. 2 1/2 Minutes.

I feel if the body is made to be very strong, really strong, it can fight off anything.

Yogi Bhajan

4
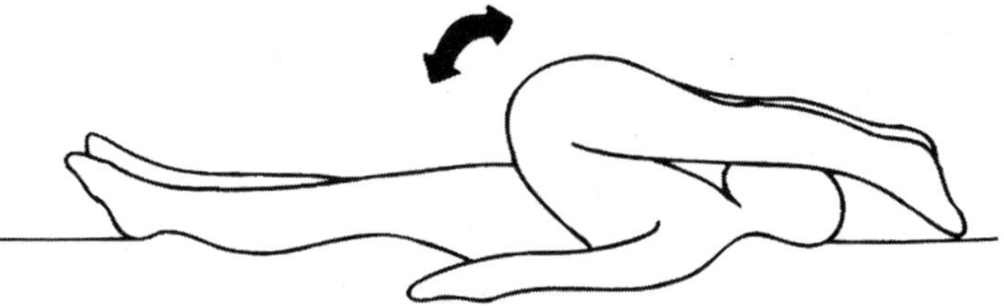

5
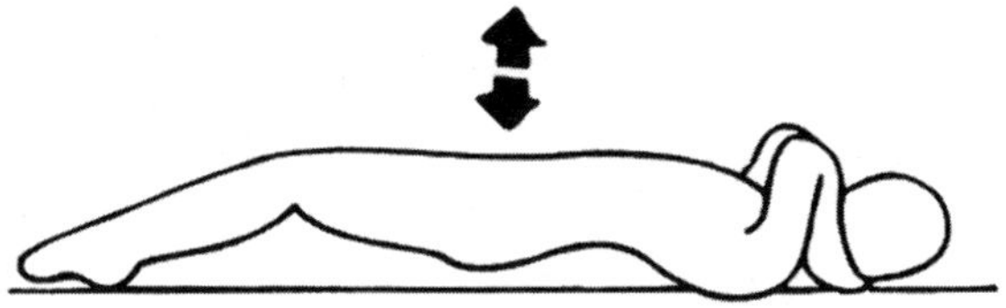

6
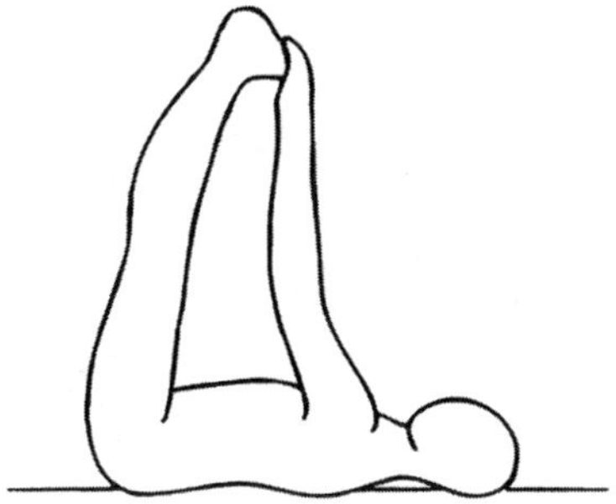

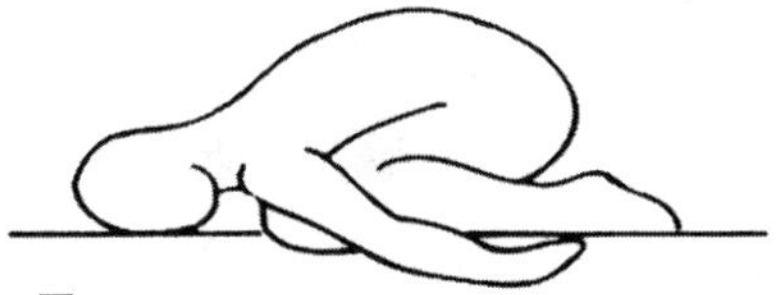
7a

7b
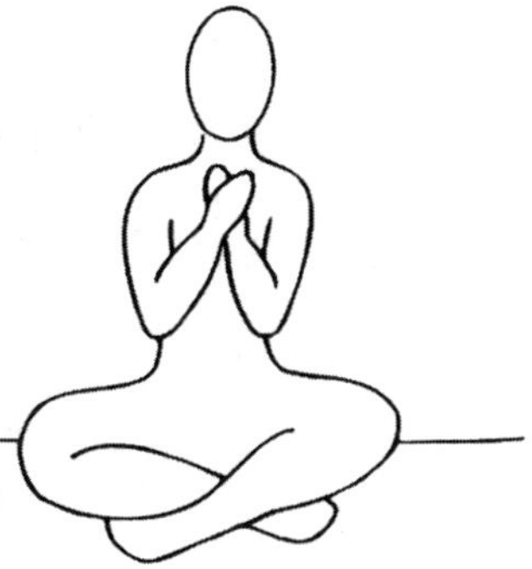

4. Lie down on your back and lift both legs up over your head into Plow Pose. Return your legs to the floor and continue leg lifts into Plow Pose. 2 Minutes.

5. Lie down straight and put your hands under your neck. Spread your heels about one foot apart. Begin jumping the body from the hips, moving from the center of the body. Don't bend the knees, but move from thighs to rib cage. Move vigorously. 3 1/2 Minutes.

6. Still lying on your back, lift your legs up, and grab your toes, keeping your knees straight. Open your mouth and breathe through your throat. 1 Minute.

7. Come into Baby Pose with your forehead on the ground and your hands behind you. Go to sleep listening to "Naad - the Blessing" by Sangeet Kaur Khalsa. After 11 Minutes rise up, cross your palms over your Heart Center and sing along with the mantra for 5 more Minutes. Yogi Bhajan played the gong during this meditation.

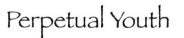

Perpetual Youth

November 20, 1990

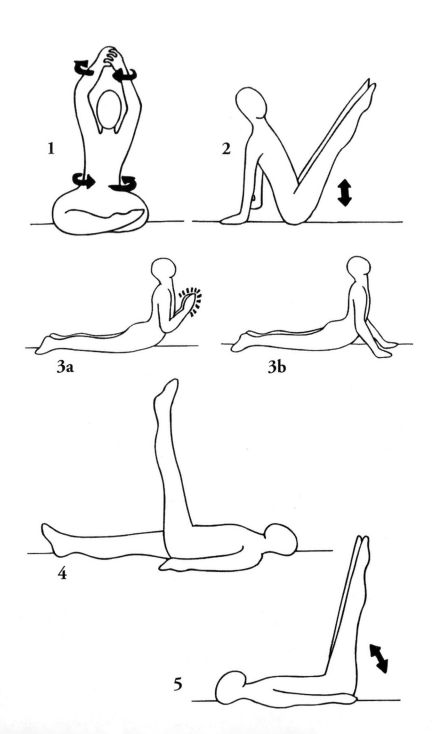

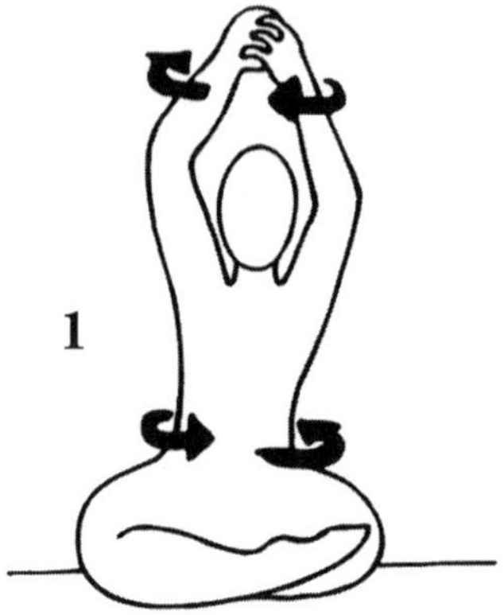

1

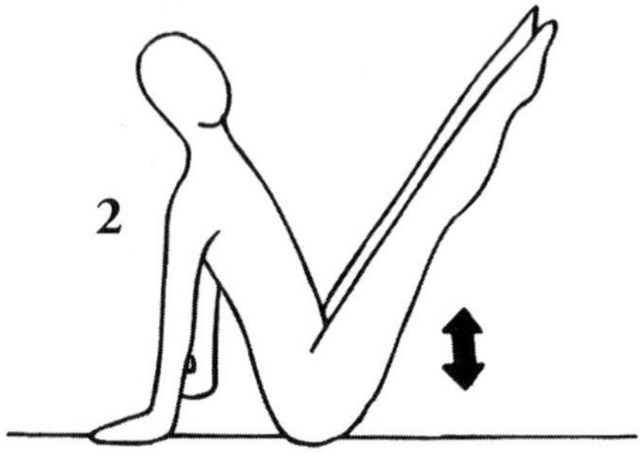

2

3a

3b

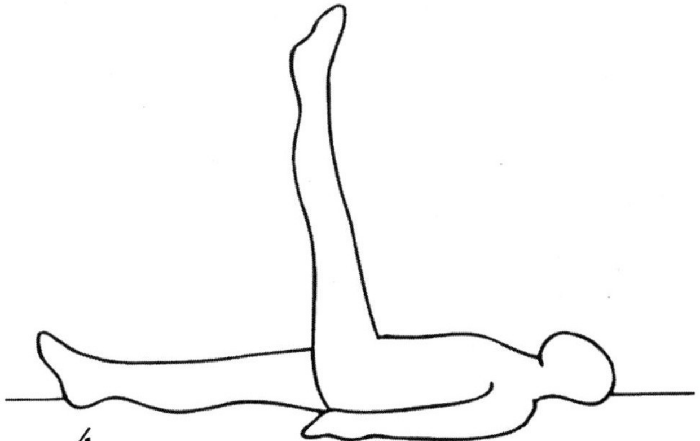

4

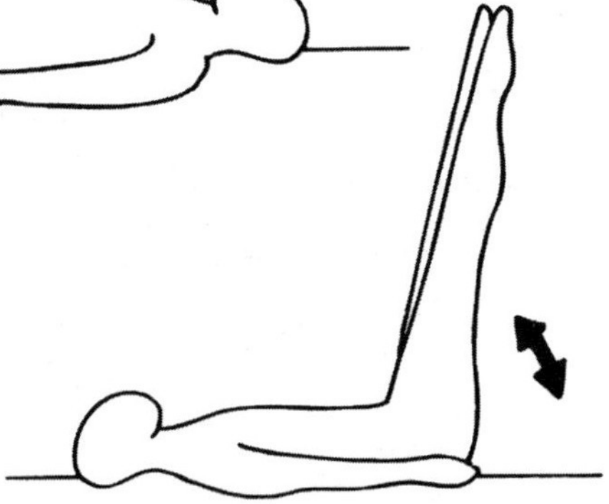

5

1. Sit in Easy Pose and lock your hands over your head in Venus Lock. Circle your midsection (grind your digestive area) counter-clockwise and circle your hands and arms in the opposite direction. Move strongly. 4 Minutes. This is good for stomach and elimination, adjusts the spine, and balances your energy.

2. Stretch your legs forward. Place your hands on the ground slightly behind you for balance. Raise both legs up and down with Breath of Fire. Time the motion with the breath. After 1 Minute, switch to long, deep breathing but continue the leg lifts. Control your movements so that the feet don't make noise when they touch the ground. 2 1/2 Minutes.

You cannot grow old if you do this exercise for 31 Minutes a day. You are balancing *prana* and *apana* by your own power. It is also good for strengthening the lower back.

3. Come into Cobra Pose. While in Cobra Pose, lift your hands off the ground, clap them together and return them to the ground. Use the strength of your spine to keep your upper body in position when your hands are off the ground. 2 Minutes.

4. Lie on your back and do alternate leg lifts up to 90°. After one minute, chant "Sa" as you lift one leg, "Ta" as you lift the other, "Na" as you lift the first leg, and "Ma" as you lift the other. Continue 2 Minutes.

5. Begin lifting both legs up to 90° together. As the legs come up, chant "Sa", as they go down, chant "Ta", as the legs come up, chant "Na" and as they go down, chant "Ma". 1 1/2 Minutes.

Three Minutes of Baby Pose adjusts gases in the body and the intestines. Many diseases come from imbalances caused by misplacements of the gross and subtle airs of the body. The subtle airs are called vayus. Adjusting all these airs prevents many ailments of old age.

Gurucharan Singh

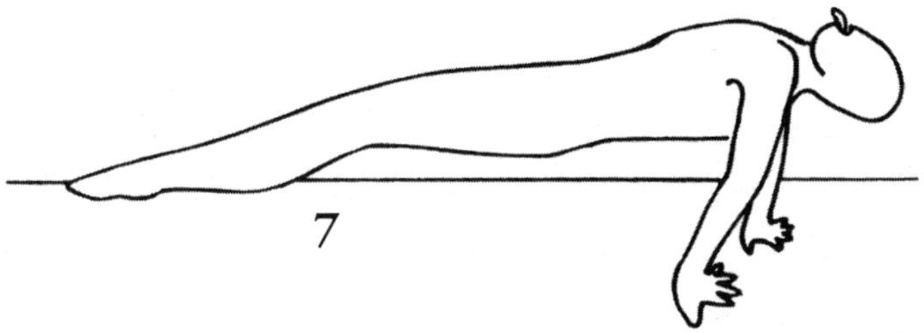

7

6. Relax. 6 Minutes.
Yogi Bhajan taught the following as a way to come out of this deep relaxation and he recommended it as the way to wake your body before you get up in the morning. Getting up too abruptly shocks your system and you can't compensate for that during the day. There is no set time for each movement,

a. Before you open your eyes in the morning, cover them with your hands and open your eyes while they are covered. Slowly bring your hands forward, uncovering your eyes so that the light comes gradually into them.
b. Cat stretch left and right.
c. Roll your neck.
d. Stretch your feet forward pointing your toes and stretch your arms up over your head.
e. Bend forward slowly and grab your toes.
f. Get into Baby Pose. Do your prayers in Baby Pose before you get up.
g. Slowly rise up and sit on your heels in rock pose.

7. Stretch your legs forward and come up into Back Platform Pose with the neck tilted back. Open your mouth, put your tongue out, and do Breath of Fire through the mouth. 1 Minute. This posture is good for the pelvis, the thyroid, and the parathyroid.

For Creativity

Circa Early 1970s

1
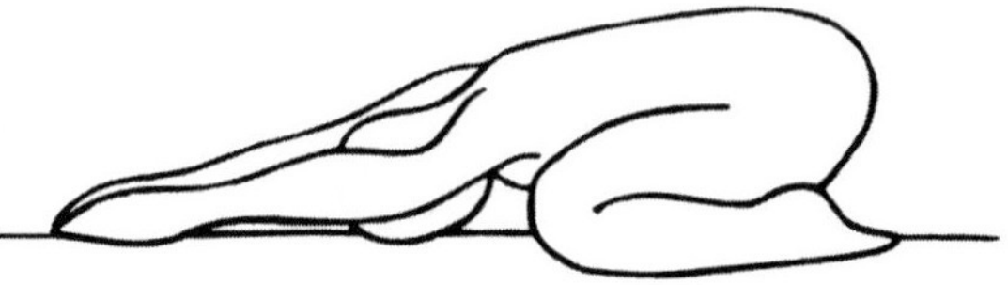

2
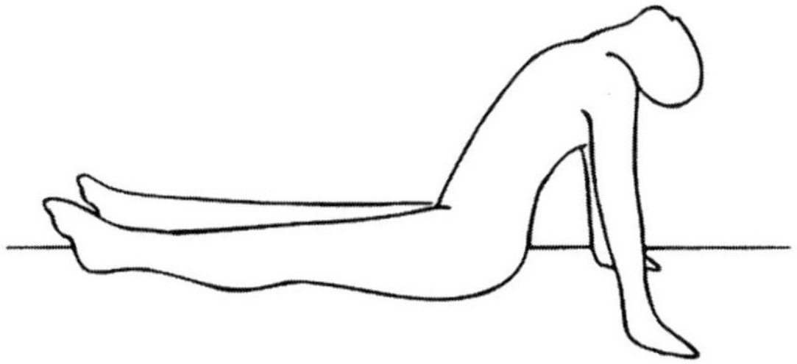

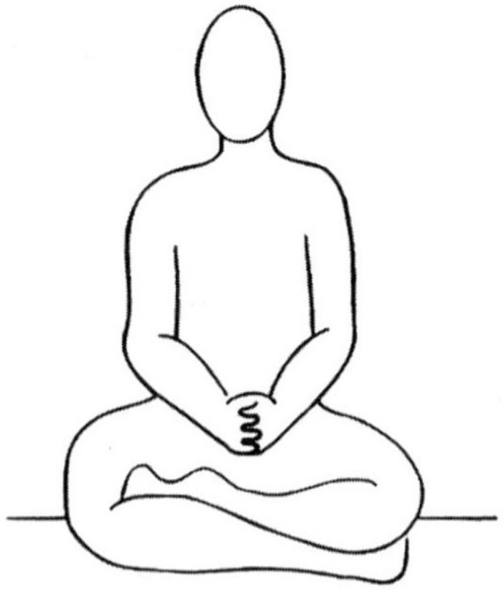
3

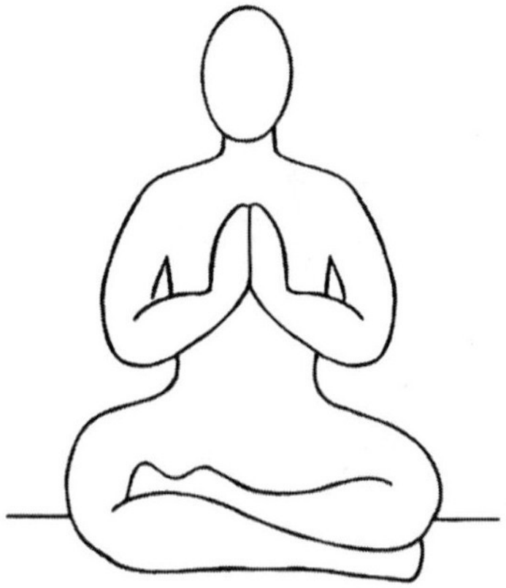
4

1. Sit on your heels, bring your forehead to the ground, arms extended forward, palms together on the ground in front of you. This position is known as *Guru Pranam* (bowing to the Teacher in all things). Inhale and mentally pull the breath energy to the base of the spine. Hold the breath and let the colors of the rainbow spread up your spine, starting with red at the base, then orange, yellow, green, blue, blue-violet and going to violet at the crown of the head. Exhale and let the colors dissolve. Inhale and begin again. Continue up to 5 Minutes.

2. Sit up, stretch your legs out straight, lean back 60° supported by your arms, and let your head fall back. Relax. A muscle block in your chest and throat will be worked out if you will breathe deeply through the nose for 3 Minutes. (The exhale must be very complete) Use the muscles of your abdomen as well as the chest muscles when breathing. On each exhale, project a beam of light out the top of your forehead. The last time, hold the breath as long as is comfortable, then sigh the air out through the nose slowly lowering yourself onto your back to relax.

3. After a short relaxation, sit up in Easy Pose, spine straight, fingers interlaced in your lap. Inhale deeply and chant the vibration *Ong* at an even pitch. Stretch the sound out as long as you can. *Ong* means the creativity of consciousness or Creative Infinity. Pull your chin in slightly, so when you sustain the "ng" sound, you can feel a vibration passing from the back part of the palate in the roof of the mouth up into the cranium gently stimulating the whole brain. This is a kind of internal massage. Continue for 11 Minutes.

4. Sit in Easy Pose and press your palms together in front of your chest, the thumbs pressing firmly on the Heart Center point. (This point is located between the fifth and sixth ribs at the center of the sternum.)
Draw your concentration there for 2 Minutes.

All art, music, poetry, dance, and handicrafts attempt to capture and reflect the flow of the universal life force. When the artist is acting sensitively, as a channel for the life force passing through him, his art gains that grace and spontaneity which touches the essence of creation. In this sense, all art is worship of God.

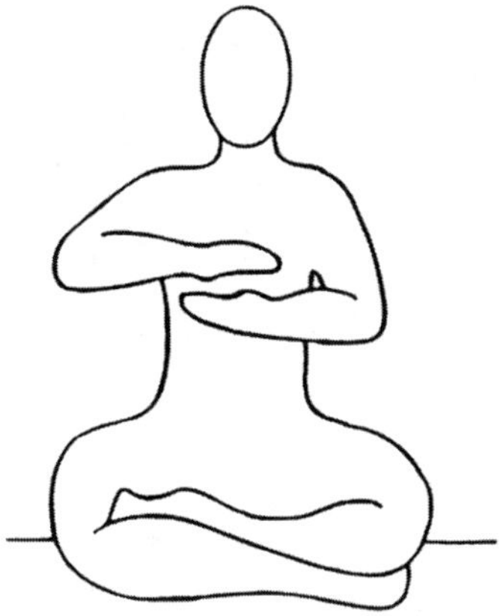

6

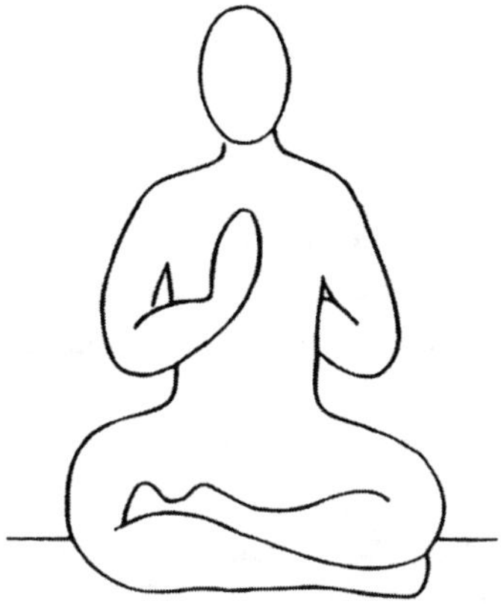

7

5. Begin rubbing your palms together vigorously, creating heat between them. Rub them for 2 Minutes, sensing the energy building up in your palms. Then draw the palms 4 inches apart, facing each other, and feel the polarity of attraction and repulsion: right palm positive, left palm negative. Close your eyes and feel the sensitivity in your palms for 2 Minutes.

6. Shift the hands so that the right hand is cupped, facing down, and left hand is cupped, facing up. They should be 4 inches apart, the Heart Center lying midway between them. Begin breathing deep and relaxed through the nostrils, gathering the breath energy between the palms, sensing it there as a glowing ball of light. Do this for 4 Minutes.

Relax into it, smile a bit; you are opening your heart. The interplay of the electromagnetic forces of the body in this meditation will act to relax those tissues in the chest and chest cavity.

7. Press your right palm firmly against the Heart Center and bring your left arm behind your back so the back of the left hand is pressed on the spine opposite the right palm. Feel the charging polarity thus set up, and begin Breath of Fire, breathing rapidly and vigorously through the nostrils, using the Navel Point as a pump. After 2 Minutes, inhale deeply and hold as long as is comfortable and exhale. Meditate quietly for a few Minutes with your spine straight and your hands in your lap, feeling Divine.

An artist takes great care of his tools, his brushes, his pen--he selects his material, his wood, clay, paper, etc. with close consideration as to what will provide the most responsive medium for his talents. Yet the fundamental tool, the mind, is left wandering, undisciplined, and full of conflicting desires. The mind is largely an unknown factor in the process of creation. It is necessary to be able to tune the mind to the basic life forces within and without, and to be able to relax the mental processes so that the spontaneous creative impulses can come through clearly and honesty.

These exercises will prove useful if they are done regularly whenever you set yourself to be creative. Creative concentration on the practice of these exercises will open the channels through which your own inner creativity can flow.

To Activate the Central Nervous System and Stimulate the Pituitary Gland

June 17, 1993

1
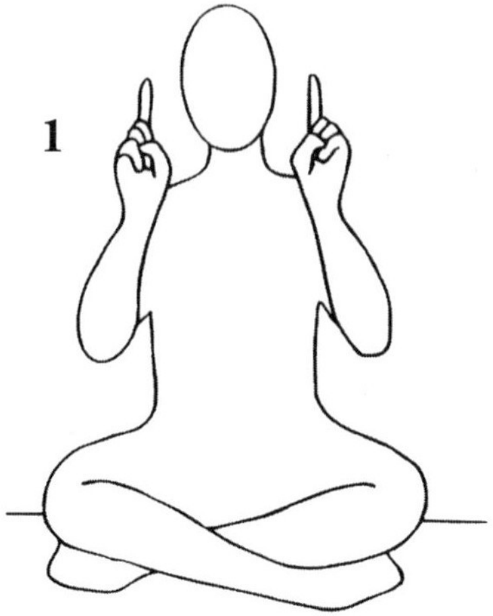

1. Sit in Easy Pose with your elbows bent and your hands a little higher than shoulder level. The index (Jupiter) finger of each hand is pointing straight upward and the other three fingers are curled into a fist with the thumb on top locking the fingers into position. Make your Jupiter fingers stiff and as hard as steel. Wrinkle your nose up so that it lifts your upper lip up from your teeth. (You will look funny.) Begin a strong breath through the tip of your nose. This is not as fast as Breath of Fire, but it must be powerful. Concentrating on the breath through the nostrils and maintaining the pressure created by wrinkling your nose will activate the *Ida* and *Pingala* energy channels. 4 Minutes.

The inner Self of the self is sitting, waiting for you to realize that Self.

Yogi Bhajan

2
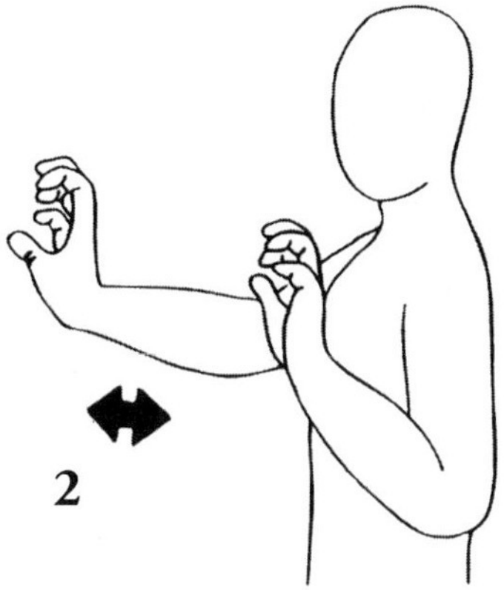

2. Sit in Easy Pose with your hands curled like lion's claws, the palms facing outward. Begin to punch with your hands fixed in this claw-like position. Form your mouth into an "O" shape and breathe in and out through the "O" shaped lips. Move quickly and the force of your punching hands will create the breath rhythm. Use this motion to release your inner anger. Be physically, mentally, and spiritually aggressive. After 2 1/2 Minutes, intensify your motion as if you really were a lion making a ferocious attack. Continue another 1 1/2 Minutes. Inhale, hold the breath, and tense the entire body, and exhale. Repeat this inhale, hold, and tense two more times. This exercise will help clear away depression.

3. Sit in Easy Pose. Stick your tongue out as far as it will go, when it reaches its maximum, clap your hands in front of your chest. Pull your tongue back in. Repeat the tongue movement and the clap. Pull your tongue in and continue. When you stretch your tongue in this manner, the little cord under the tongue is pulled and that pull stimulates the central nervous system, which is the control center of your life. 3 Minutes. Inhale, stick the tongue out to the maximum, hold the breath for 10 seconds, and exhale. Repeat this two more times to complete the exercise.

This exercise has a progressive and gradual impact on the nervous system. Most people experience this sequence of nervous system signposts: after you do it 3 or 4 times the back of the tongue will start hurting, then the tongue will hurt on both sides, and then, after 3 Minutes, the neurons in your head will start changing and you will feel fine.

Gurucharan Singh

4
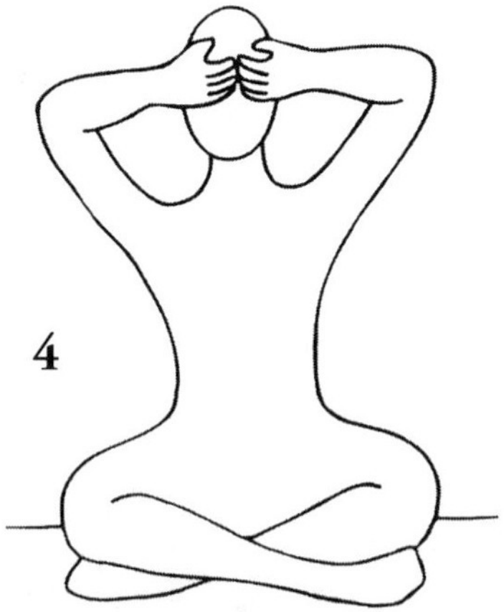

4. Sit in Easy Pose and place both hands on your forehead with all eight fingers touching the forehead. The elbows are out to the sides up almost at the level of the forehead. Close your eyes, become calm, and sing along with the chanting from Wahe Guru Kaur's "Aquarian Sadhana." 18 Minutes.
Inhale, concentrate on the point between the eyebrows at the root of the nose, bringing all your energy there, and exhale. Repeat this two more times to complete the exercise.
After you have done this set, do not drink alcohol or coffee or in any way stimulate yourself. Rest and preserve the energy you have created. It will heal your body very much.

For Inner Vitality and Stamina

Spring, 1992

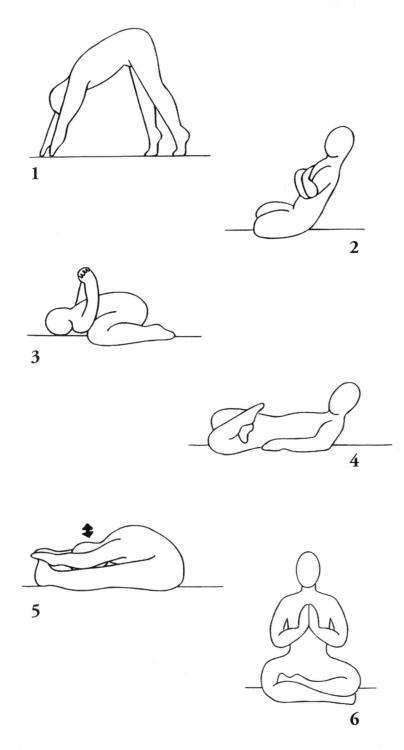

1

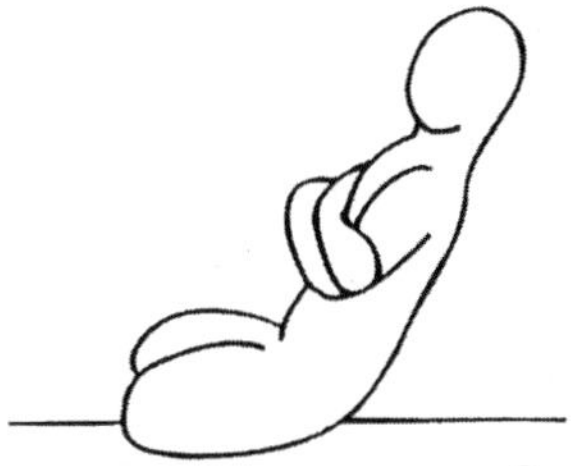

2

3

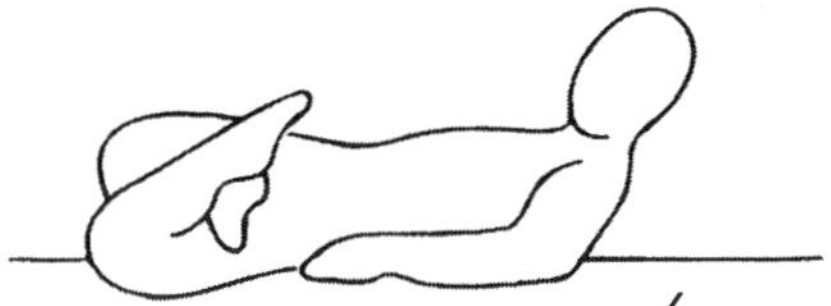

4

5

6

1. Balance on your toes and fingertips with the knees straight but not locked. Rapidly move your hips from side to side like an animal swishing its tail. 3 Minutes

2. Sitting in Easy Pose, lean back to 60°. Fold your arms across your chest and lock your elbows with your hands at diaphragm level. Keep your neck straight with your chin pulled in and roll your shoulders in a forward circle. 3 Minutes

3. Come into Baby Pose. Bring both hands to the small of your back and interlock your fingers. Raise your arms up into Yoga Mudra. 3 Minutes.

4. Cross your legs in Lotus Pose and lean back on your elbows. 3 Minutes.

5. Stretch your legs out in front of you and grab your toes. Bring your head to your knees and come back up. Do this movement rapidly 11 times only. Breathe normally, do not do Breath of Fire.

6. Sit in Easy Pose, with your hands in Prayer Pose at the center of your chest. Focus your eyes at the tip of your nose. Keep your chin in, chest out and neck straight. Pump your Navel Point and imagine 30 trillion points of light in and around you. 3 Minutes.

To finish: inhale deeply, hold your breath and tighten every muscle of your body. Hold the breath for 10 seconds and then let it go out of the mouth explosively like cannon fire. Repeat this 2 more times.

This set takes only fifteen minutes and it can make you a Miracle Kid. You can become a successful Aquarian person.

Immune Yoga I

January 30, 1990

1 & 2

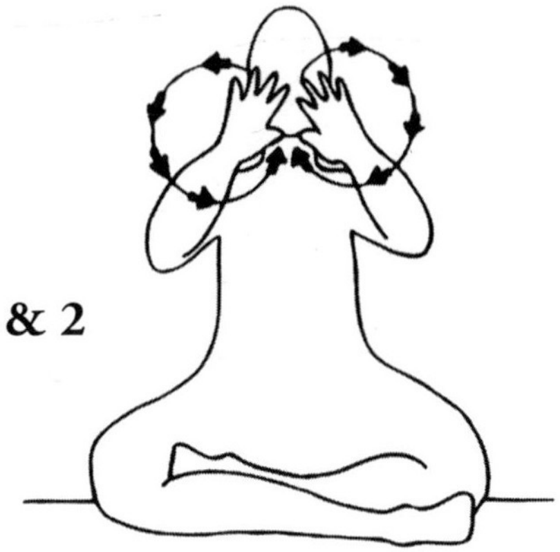

1. Sit in Easy Pose. The elbows are bent and the arms are at the sides palms facing forward. The hands are about the level of the ears. The fingers are spread. Begin rapidly moving your hands in small outward circles. These circles pass in front of the face and body as if you were using both hands to wipe a mirror in front of you. The movement is so vigorous that the buttocks are pulled a little off the ground during the circling. Keep your eyes open during this exercise. 5 1/2 Minutes. This exercise works on the thymus gland, the gland which controls all blood diseases. It promotes good circulation in the breast area. The area around the collarbone and the shoulders will be worked on and will feel the effects of the movement.

Relax 1-2 Minutes, but don't close your eyes. If your vision becomes fuzzy, drink a glass of water.

3

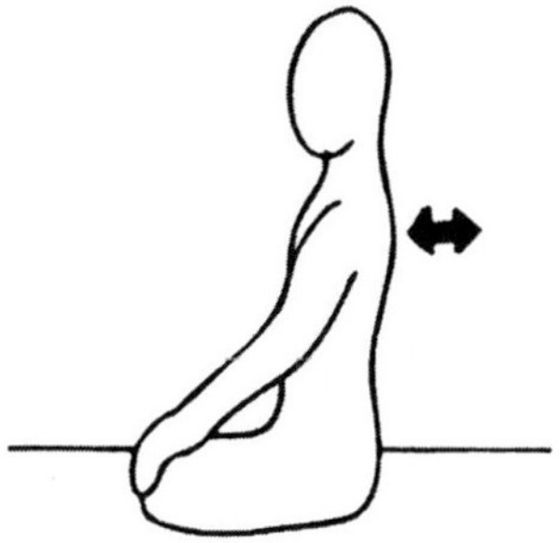

2. Bend your neck forward and press your chin against your chest and repeat exercise 1 for 2 1/2 Minutes. This exercise moves the parathyroid physically. A healthy parathyroid keeps us young; we get old because the parathyroid does not support our thyroid. Bending the neck forward in this way puts pressure on the thyroid and parathyroid. (Please note that this is not our standard form of Jalandhara Bandh, but a variation of it.) Relax for 1 Minute. Keep your eyes open and stay alert.

3. Still in Easy Pose, put your hands on your knees (hands cup around the knees comfortably). Using the strength of your hands begin a spinal flex of the area between your shoulder blades. 4 Minutes. Relax but keep your eyes open for 1 Minute.

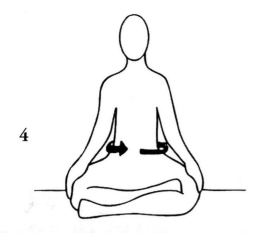

4

4. Sitting in the same position as Exercise 3, begin churning your digestive area, moving counter-clockwise. Churn powerfully to move the lower vertebra next to the tailbone. 4 1/2 Minutes. This will give your muscles a new blood supply. The major glandular system is controlled by the pelvic bone area and this adjusts that area.

I am not a person who believes in catering to students, but I do cater to the honesty of the teaching. I learned as a good student. I teach as a good student to a good student. That is the Master's way.

Yogi Bhajan

7 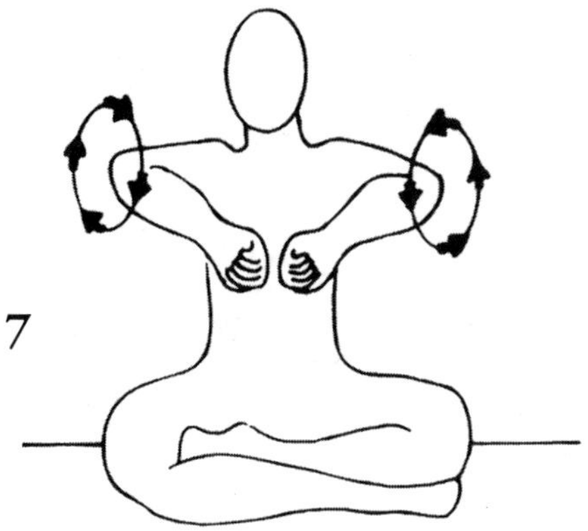

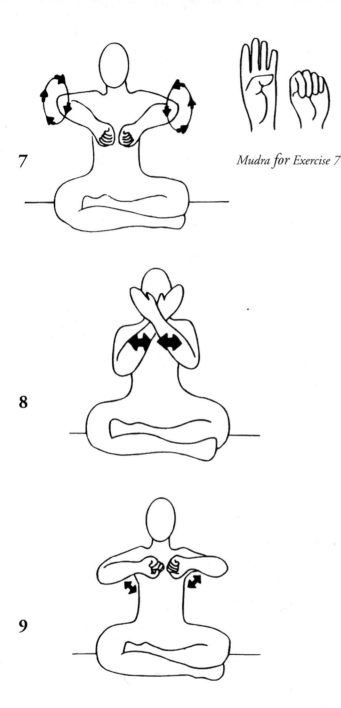

Mudra for Exercise 7

8 

9 

5. Roll your hands around your wrists for 30 seconds. Relax 5 Minutes. Either sit or walk around. Keep your eyes open, don't be sleepy, stay alert, and talk. Take this time to let the glandular secretion penetrate into the body.

6. Sitting again in Easy Pose with your hands on your knees, begin pumping your navel in and out. Breathe normally. Keep your eyes open.
6 1/2 Minutes.

7. Touch your thumbs to the mound of the Mercury (little) finger and make a fist. Raise your bent elbows, with your fists in front of your chest. Circle the elbows forward. 2 Minutes. This stimulates the magnetic area of the heart.

8. Criss-cross your forearms and hands rapidly in front of your face. Look straight ahead. The fingers are together with the thumbs pressed in and the palms are facing towards you. The right hand is nearest the body. Lean backward a little bit. Move fast. This is for the nervous system. 2 Minutes.

9. Beat your elbows and upper arms against your rib cage (like chicken wings). The hands are in fists. The armpits are the center of the nervous system and must move during this exercise. The arms hit the rib cage rapidly and hard. This will make you young. 3 Minutes.

Break: Stand up and go for a walk. You cannot sit. You must allow the system to absorb the energy. 5 Minutes.

10. Sit in Easy Pose. Stick out your tongue and do Breath of Fire through your mouth. 1 Minute.

To finish: Inhale, hold the breath 20 seconds, tighten the body and exhale. You must send the energy to the entire body. Do this two more times.

The Navel Point is the source of the reserve energy that initiates the Kundalini energy to awaken and flow. It is the source of your real inner strength.

Gurucharan Singh

Immune Yoga II

January 31, 1990

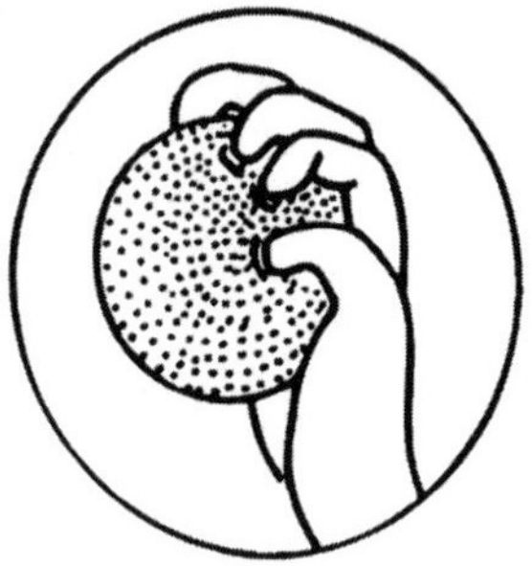

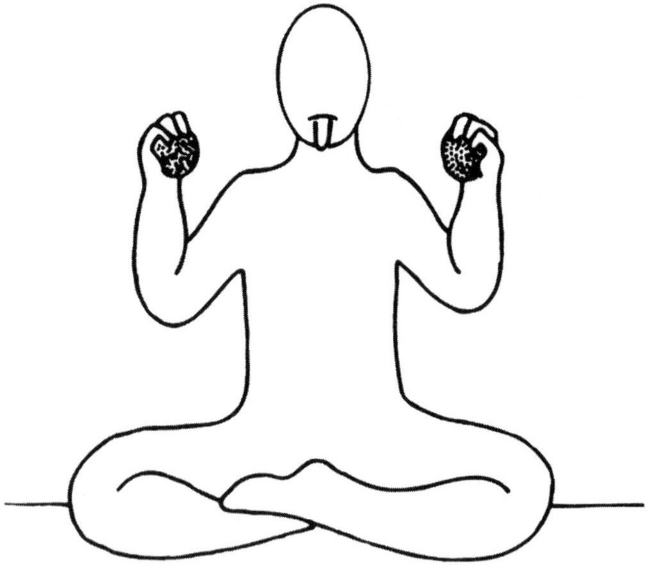

You will need 2 oranges.

1. Sitting in Easy Pose, hold one orange in each hand. Dig your five fingernails into the orange as if you were holding it in a lion's claws. Your elbows are bent, palms are facing each other, holding the oranges up above shoulder level. Your eyes are on the tip of your nose and the tongue is out. Grasp your oranges tightly with your fingernails, really dig them in. The fingers are the antennae of the five parts of the brain and represent the left and right hemispheres. Play "Rakhe Rakhanhar" by Nirinjan Kaur very softly. Keep the posture and stay steady. 17 Minutes.

Inhale and exhale. Shake your hands over your head. 1/2 Minute.
Walk and talk and move around the room, but do not close your eyes.

11 Minutes.

2. Sit down again holding the oranges as in exercise 1. Eyes are at the tip of your nose and the tongue is fully extended out of the mouth. Play "Rakhe Rakhanhar" more loudly this time. 14 Minutes.

Relax. Shake your hands and jump all around to move the energy everywhere in the body. Peel your oranges and eat them.

3. Sit in Easy Pose. Look upwards toward the sky and laugh as loud as you can. 1 Minute. Inhale and relax.

The key to this exercise is the connection between the fingers and the five elements. The five elements and the five parts of the brain within each hemisphere correspond. They stimulate the brain to release old problems and emotions and finally achieve a new integration and balance.

Gurucharan Singh

This is a very powerful re-birthing experience. You will touch your anger at the time of birth. It will reduce your inner anger, which totally controls your mood. As you do this kriya, allow your body to go through its changes: if you cough, sneeze, or cry, just go through it. Let it out naturally, consciously.

Yogi Bhajan

For Energy and Rejuvenation

April 4,1992

This set is to be done at the bathroom sink or someplace where you have a bar or a support to hold on to.

1 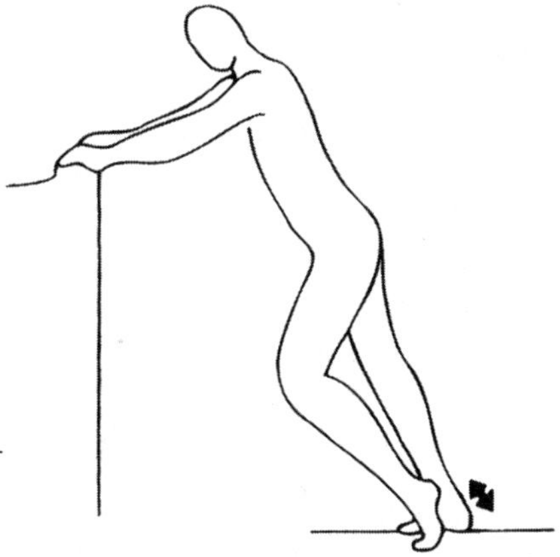

1. Grab the edge of a sink and, using it for support, walk your feet backwards until you are holding your body at a 45 degree slope from heels to head. You will feel a stretch in your hamstrings. Begin raising and lowering alternate heels, walking in place without lifting the toes off the ground. Your arms and legs are fully extended and the body bends slightly in the middle. As you walk, you may lower your head, it does not have to be held up. Walk vigorously and work up a sweat. 11 Minutes.

This set keeps one absolutely healthy, keeps the metabolism moving for the day, and keeps one in shape.

Yogi Bhajan

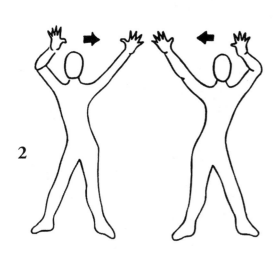

2 

2. Stand with your feet shoulder width apart and extend your arms above your head with the palms facing forward, the elbows slightly bent, and the fingers spread wide apart. Swing your arms from side to side, keeping the hands above shoulder level. The momentum of the arm swing will cause the hips to swing if you are doing the movement with enough force. Continue 11 Minutes

3 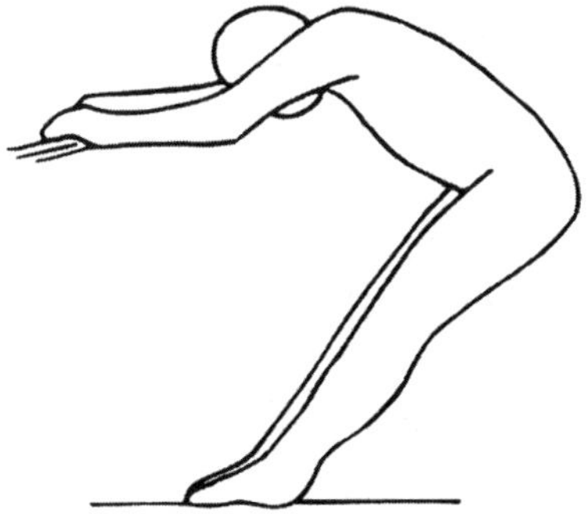

3. Once again grab the edge of the sink. Bend at the waist with your head down between your arms. You will feel a stretch in your lower back and in the backs of your legs. Relax and stretch for 11 Minutes.

Yoga for Children

August 1991

Two exercises must be done with a partner.

1. Sit in Rock Pose with your hands in Venus Lock behind your back. Open your mouth and stick your tongue out as far as you can. Inhale in the up position and, as you exhale, bring your forehead to the ground, keeping your mouth open and your tongue out. This exercise corrects imbalances in the reproductive system.

2. Sit in Celibate Pose with your hands in Venus Lock on the top of your head. Inhale and twist left. Exhale and twist right. This exercise balances the glandular system. If it is painful to sit in Celibate Pose, it is an indication that the glandular system may be out of balance.

3. Sit in Easy Pose, back to back with a partner. Cross your hands over your heart (right on top of left) and press them tightly against your chest. Bend forward and touch your forehead to the ground and come sitting up straight and hit your back and spine against your partner's spine. Continue at a steady pace and be careful not to hit heads with your partner. This exercise adjusts the spine.

4. Sit in Easy Pose, facing your partner. Put your hands around each other's neck with your arms straight and begin grinding your spine in a circular motion together with your partner. This exercise corrects menstrual problems and balances the sex glands. It also helps to keep the breast area healthy.

It is easier to prevent ill health than it is to correct an unhealthy condition once it has established itself. This set strengthens and balances children's bodies to prepare them to face adolescence and adulthood.

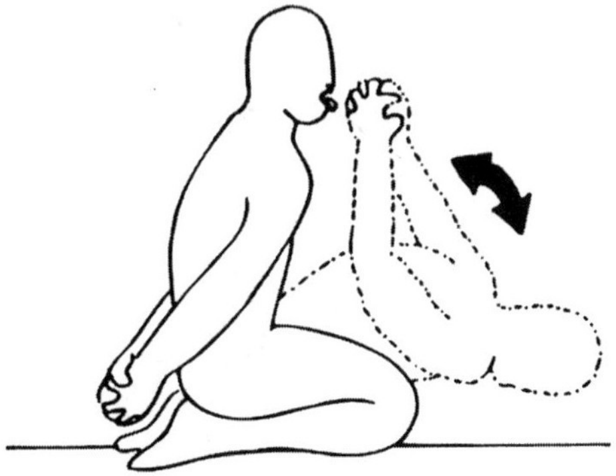

1

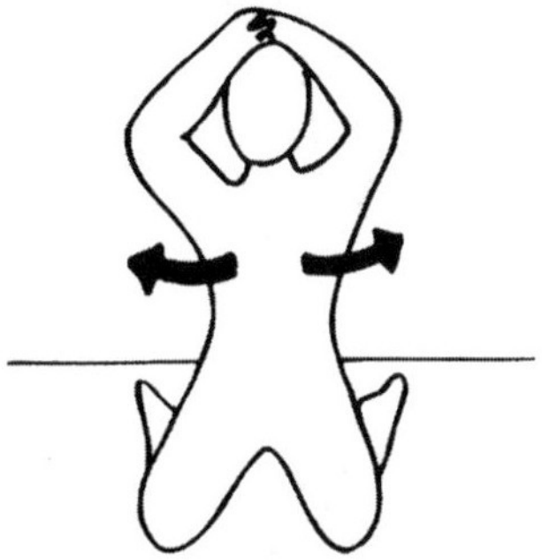

2

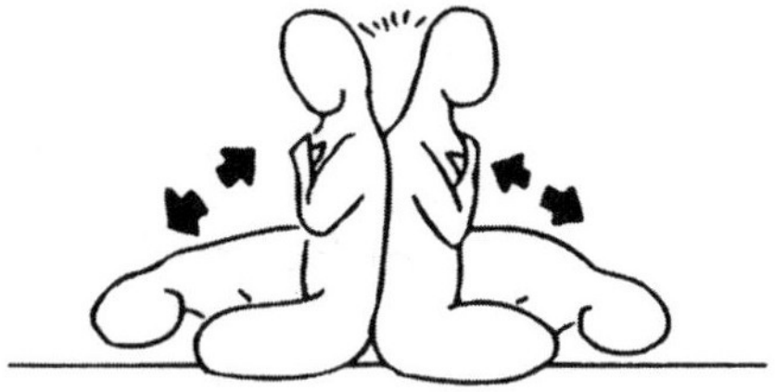

3

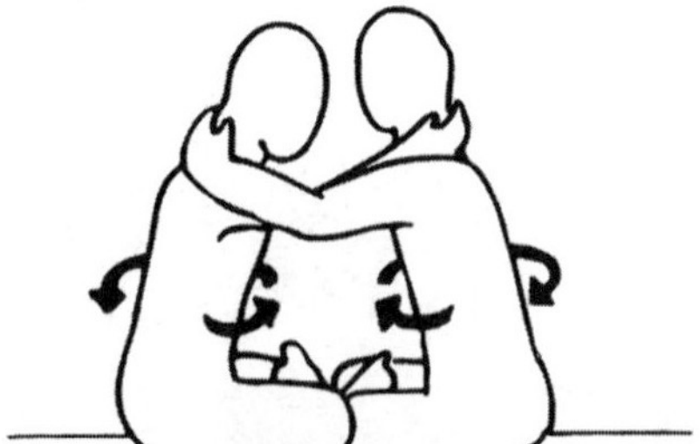

4

5
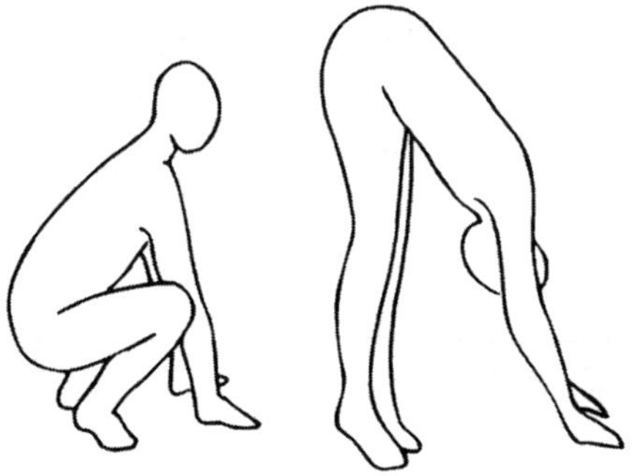

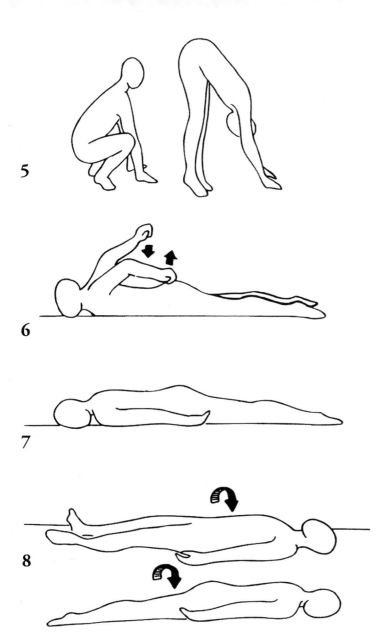

6
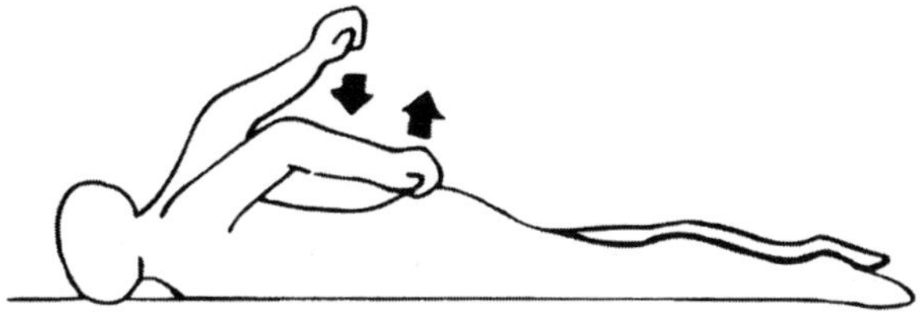

7

8
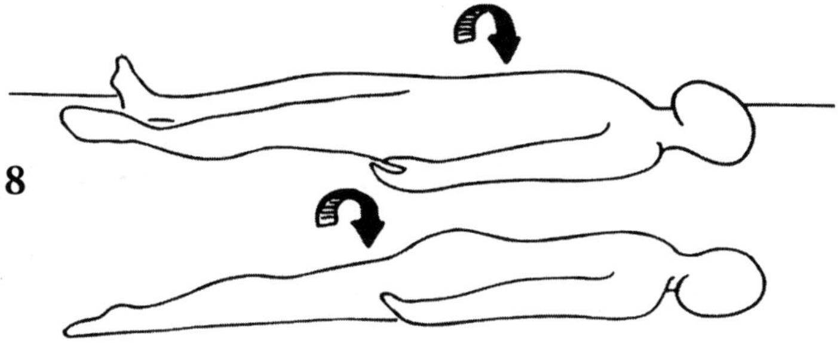

5. Frog Pose, inhaling up and exhaling down 52 times. This exercise stretches the Life Nerve and transmutes sexual energy.

6. Lie on your stomach with your chin on the ground. Make fists of your hands and beat them against your buttocks. Do this as hard and fast as you can. This exercise is very relaxing.

7. Stay on your stomach, turn your cheek to the side and fall asleep. Pretend you are sleeping and snore. Whoever does this will not snore at night.

8. Bundle Roll. Bring your arms to your sides and lock them there. Do not bend your arms or legs. Become like a log and roll, first one direction and then the other. Repeat 7 or 8 times in each direction. This exercise will break down anything in your body that shouldn't be growing and readjust the magnetic field.

There are no set times for these exercises. Do them as long as the children have attention span to participate in them. (Adults doing this set can do each exercise for 3-5 Minutes.) When teaching yoga to children, invoke their imaginations. Create a story or ask them to pretend to be animals--whatever it takes to create an imaginary environment in which the children can participate with enthusiasm and abandon.

Yoga for Young People

December 31, 1988

1

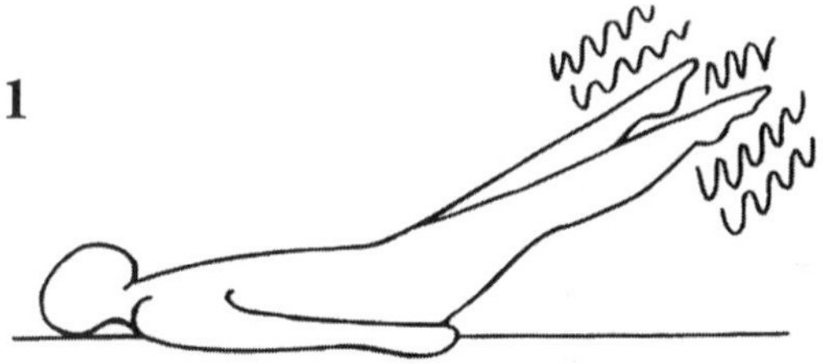

2

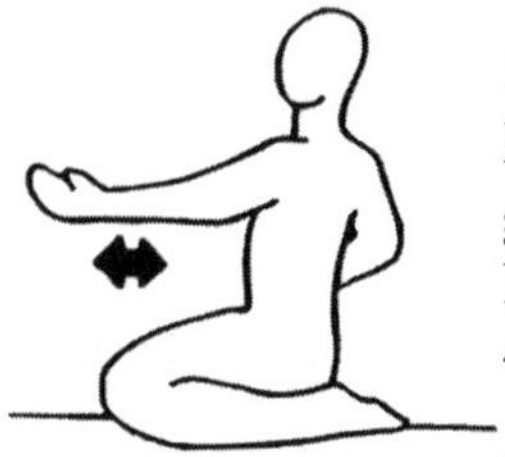

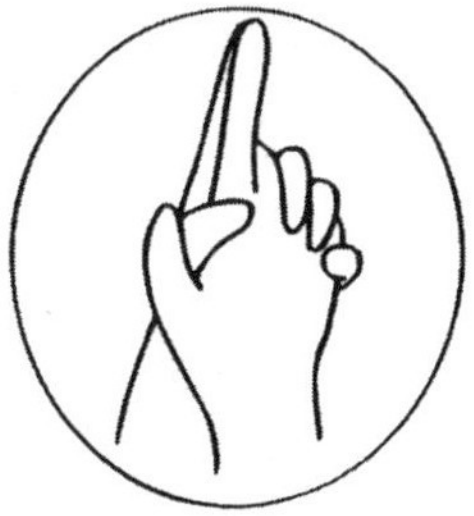

mudra for exercise 3b

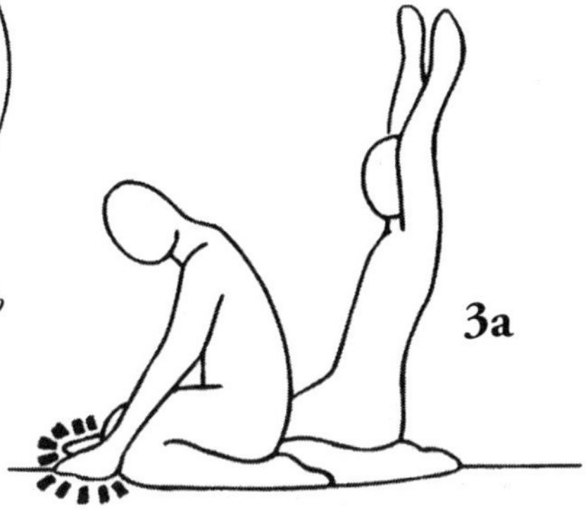

3a

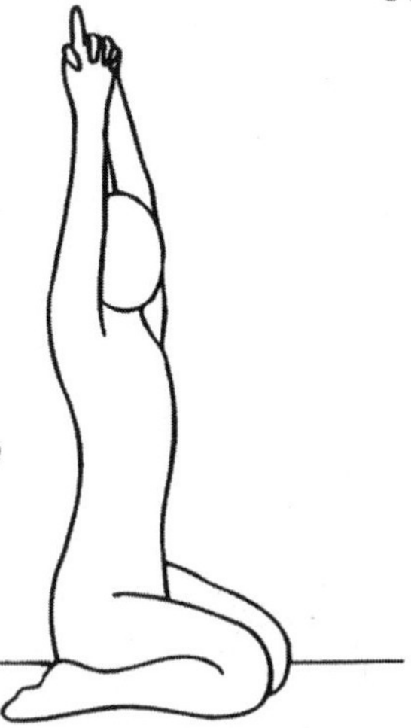

3b

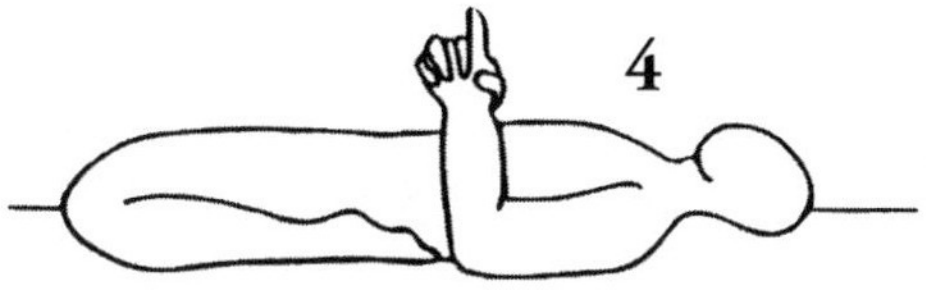

4

1. Lie down on your back and lift both legs up to 30°. Shake your feet and legs—make your feet dance. Your knee and ankle joints shake but the legs are generally straight. Breathe deeply, shake in rhythm, and chant along with Nirinjan Kaur and Guru Prem Singh's "Har Har Har Har Gobinde." 4 1/2 Minutes.

(As a stand-alone exercise to develop invincible stamina: Lie on your back and lift both legs up to 30°. Shake your feet and legs, making them dance, breathe deeply and chant anything you want for 31 Minutes.)

2. Sit in Celibate Pose. (First sit on your heels, then spread your heels apart until your buttocks are resting on the floor between your legs.) Extend your arms with the hands slightly cupped, as if you were lightly holding something very precious in each hand. Begin pushing out your right arm as you pull back your left arm. The arm motion is almost like a punch, one arm moves out as the other pulls back. Let your body move left and right at the waist with the punching motion. Close your eyes and chant along with the same mantra as in Exercise 1 for 2 Minutes.

3a. Stay in Celibate Pose. Raise the arms straight up over your head and then bring them palms down to hit the ground on either side of your knees. Raise your arms straight up and continue. Hit the ground with great force, using your whole body weight. Move to the rhythm of "Har Singh, Nar Singh, Neel Narayan" by Nirinjan Kaur. 1 minute.

3b. Then raise arms overhead, join them with the palms together with the Jupiter (index) finger extended and the other fingers locked over each other (as in beginner's Sat Kriya). Sit quietly and meditate on the music. Keep the spine pulled up and the arms straight. After 1 minute begin to chant loudly from the Navel Point. Continue chanting for 3 Minutes.

4. Lie back with the legs still in Celibate Pose, but with the back on the floor. The hands are in the same mudra as in exercise 3 but now it is placed at the Navel Point, with the Index finger pointing straight up.

There is a very powerful psychic power under the Navel Point. It sits there like a cobra snake and when it wakes up, it travels through the six centers of the body and awakens them with its touch. When it touches the seventh center, the man knows all. When it ingle-mingles with the aura, it delightfully enlightens the arc line and makes everything work out for the person.

Yogi Bhajan

Continue to chant along with the mantra for 3 Minutes.
If you cannot do this posture, there is dis-ease in your body.

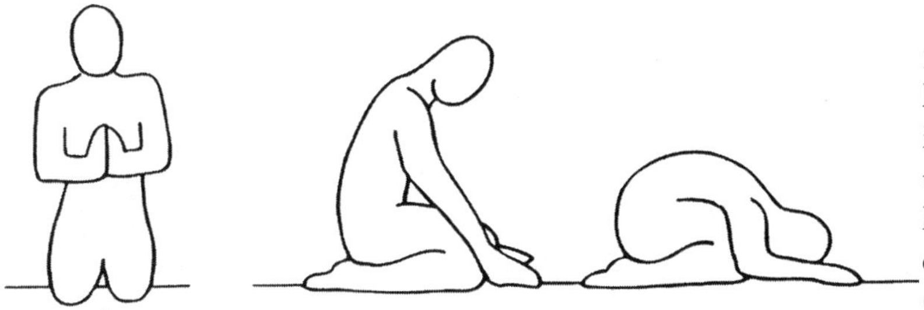

5 *Intro* 5a 5b

5. This exercise is done with Ragi Sat Nam Singh's *Jaap Sahib.* Sit on your heels with your hands in Prayer Pose in the center of your chest during the introductory prayer (about 45 seconds). Sing from your Heart Center. When the ragi sings the lines that begin with "Namastang" or "Namo", bow your head down to the floor and rise up again. Your hands are on the floor on either side of your knees. Stop at "Cha chri Chand" 3 3/4 Minutes.
(Even if you don't know the words, listen and try to chant along with the mantra.)

When the Mughals conquered India, they destroyed the entire literature of yoga, because they so feared the capacity of yoga to make people unconquerable.

Yogi Bhajan

6. Hans (Swan) Kriya

This kriya opens up the spine and invigorates the spinal serum, improves the quality of the blood, and rejuvenates the grey matter of the brain. It refreshes the capillaries, builds strength in the body and keeps the heart in good condition.

Sit on your heels with your hands on the floor on either side of your knees. Round the spine outward (which pulls the chin into the chest and rounds the back of the neck) and bow your head to the floor. Put the total weight of your upper body on the tops of your thighs as your head bows down. From this position arch your back and neck as in Cobra Pose, rising up into a sitting position and begin rounding your spine outward again. The movement is an undulation of the spine: rounding, arching, and stretching. Do this

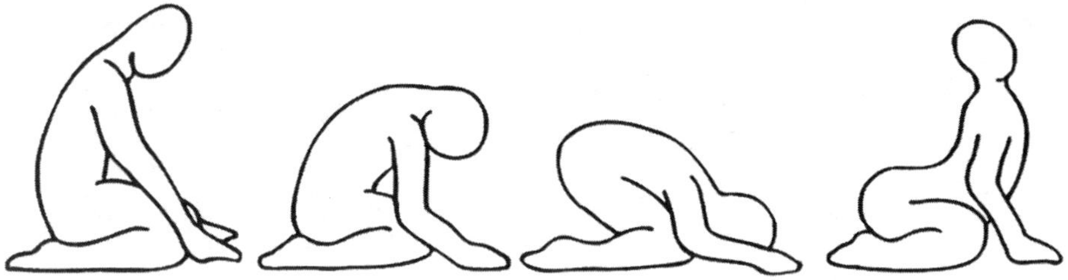

6a 6b 6c 6d

More Yoga for Young People

December 1988

1. Four Corner Lotus to adjust the navel: lying on your back, raise your arms and legs off the ground. Spread all four limbs wide open and stretch. You will be balancing on your lower back. 1 minute.

2. Sit in Baby Pose and from there rise up into Camel Pose. Stay in Camel Pose and chant loudly with Nirinjan Kaur and Guru Prem Singh's "Har Har Har Har Gobinde." 2-3 Minutes.

3. Meditation to develop unconquerable spirit: Sit in Easy Pose, with the hands in Prayer Pose at the center of the chest. The thumbs are locked. Sit with a straight spine, the lower back is lifted and stretched slightly. Close your eyes and look at the tip of your nose through the closed eyelids. Chant along with Bhai Avtar Singh and Bhai Gurucharan Singh's "Jai Te Gang" pulling the Navel Point in with each repetition of the word "Jai". Continue 3 to 62 Minutes.

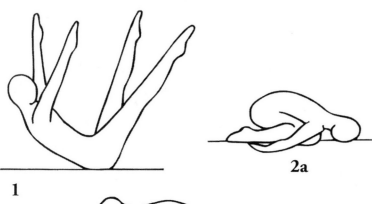

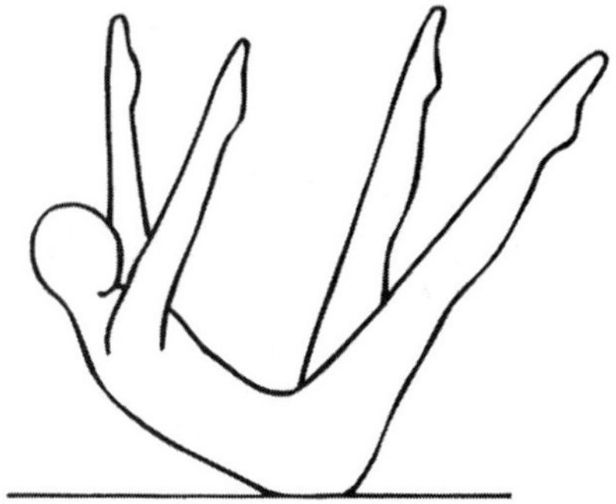

1

2a

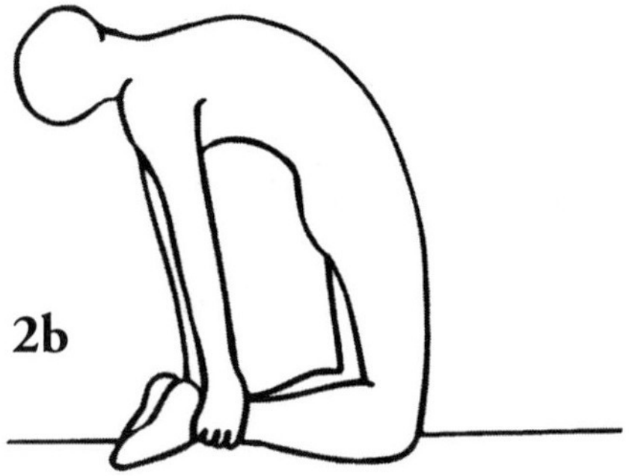

2b

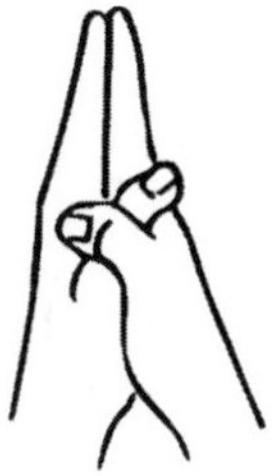

Mudra for Exercise 3

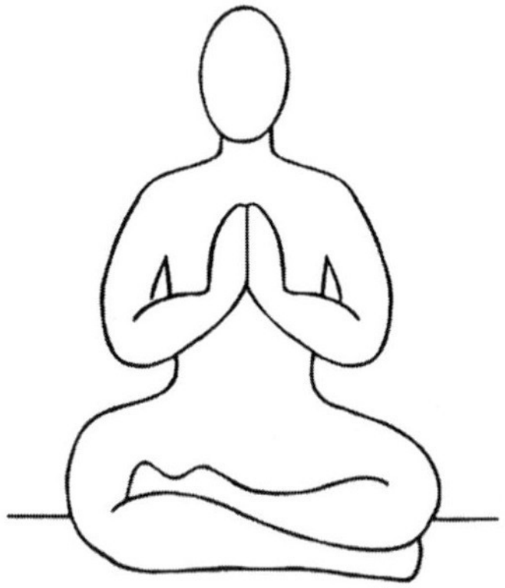

3

If you can perfect Camel Pose in childhood, in old age you will have no extra fat on the body. To perfect this posture means that you can stay in it for 31 Minutes. Start with two to three Minutes then slowly and gradually increase the time.

If you know "Jai Te Gang" perfectly by heart and can meditate on it at your Navel Point, nobody can conquer you: no enemy, no friend, no god, no demon, no angel, nobody.

Yogi Bhajan

Wake Up, Warm Up, and Get Up

Simple Things to Do Before You Get Up in the Morning

March 1992

This routine is very helpful on those days when you have to get up and you don't want to.

If, before getting up and before opening your eyes, you spend one minute doing the following things, you will preserve your health and prevent disease.

1. Clench your fingers.
2. Move your shoulders in a circle.
3. Tense and release your lower back.
4. Point your toes.
5. With your hands flat at your sides, stretch your whole body.
6. Curl around sinuously like a snake, 3 inches left and right.
7. Put the palms of your hands over your eyes, open your eyes while your hands are covering them, and then slowly move your hands forward and away from your eyes. In this way your eyes become gently introduced to the first light of day.
8. Massage your mouth and face with the palms of both hands.
9. Cat stretch left and right.
10. Raise your head up slowly and pull your knees up to your chest.

Now get up and enjoy your day.

Re-vibrate the Immune System

June 2, 1986

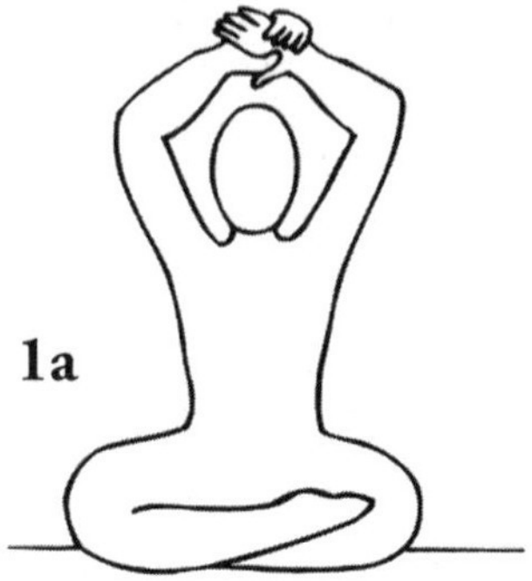
1a

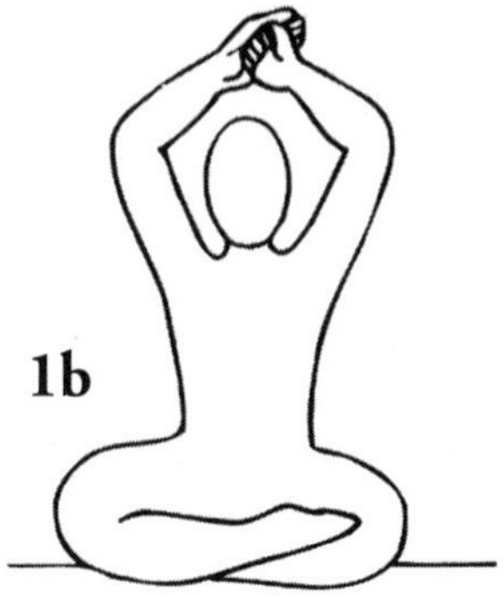
1b

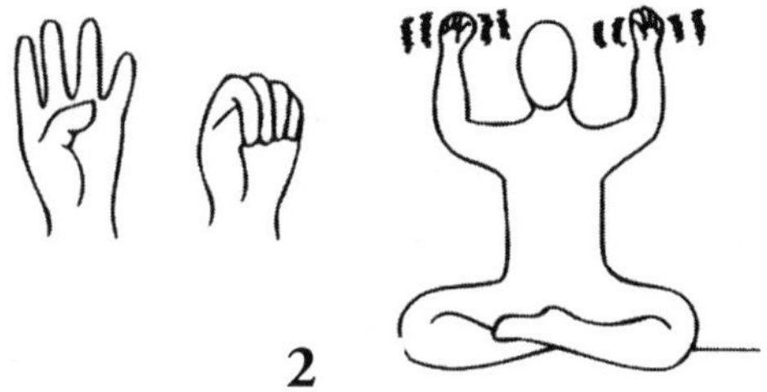
2

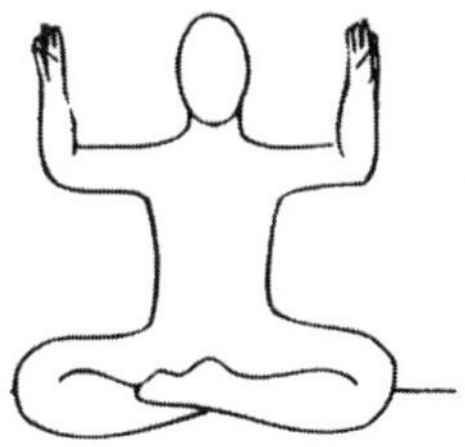
4a

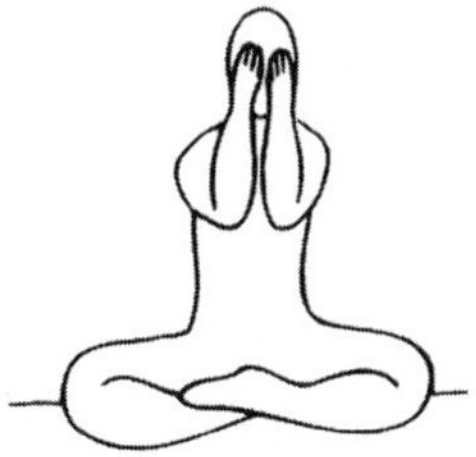
4b

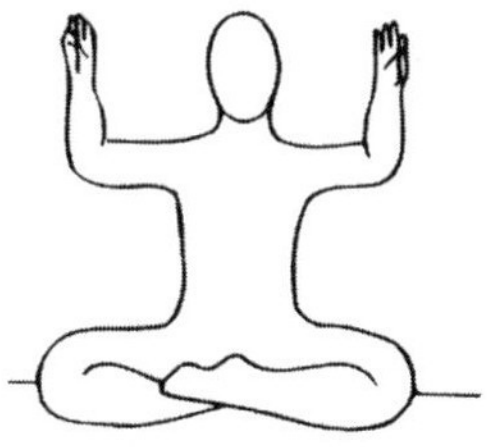
4c

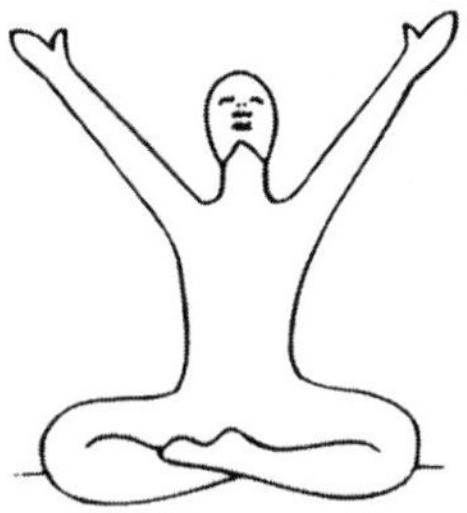
5

You will need a mixture of 9 parts pineapple juice and 1 part coconut juice for this set. Have 8 to 12 oz. available for each of the two times when you are required to drink your juice.

1. Raise your hands above your head, palms facing forward. Place the right palm against the back of the left hand with the thumbs crossed so that the right thumb is in front of the left. Grip the back of the left hand with the right hand. Then grip the right thumb with the left hand. Continue this action, alternating the grips rhythmically. Make a circle of your lips and breathe strongly and deeply through the mouth. Inhale and grip with one hand. Exhale and grip with the other hand. 10 Minutes.

2. Place your thumbs on the mound of the Sun finger (ring finger) and close the fist around the thumb. Hold your fists on either side of your head. Inhale and hold your breath for 20 seconds while shaking your hands rapidly and powerfully. Exhale. Do this inhale-hold-and-shake a total of seven times.

This movement will totally revitalize you if you really do it hard. Do it with such strength that your buttocks move to keep your balance during the shaking.

3. Drink 8 to 12 oz. of your juice. Relax 3 Minutes.

4. Panj Mudra: hold your arms out to the sides. The elbows are bent with the forearms and fingers pointing upwards. The arms are pulled back so that the forearms are a little behind the ears. The hands are about the level of the eyes. Touch your thumb and Mercury (little) finger and bring your hands and forearms in front of your face and then return back to the first position. Release the mudra. Touch your thumb and Sun (ring) finger and bring your hands and forearms in front of your face then return back to the first position at the sides. Release the mudra. Touch your thumb and Saturn (middle) finger and bring your hands and forearms in front of your face then return back to the sides. Release the mudra. Touch your thumb and Jupiter (pointer) finger and bring your hands and forearms in front of

We have two strengths: the life force and the re-creative strength of the life force which is within us.

Yogi Bhajan

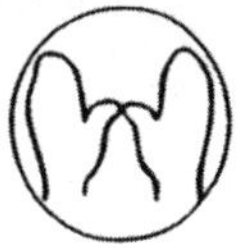

Hand Position for Exercise 6

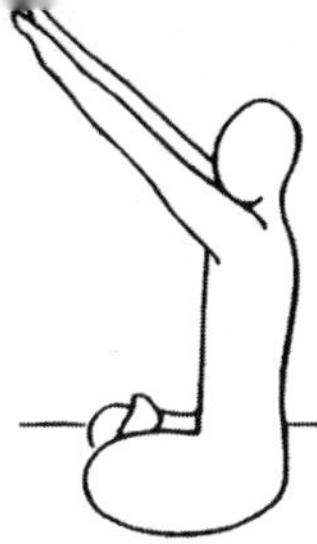

6

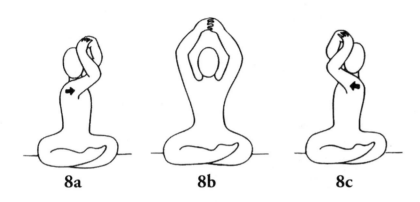

8a

8b

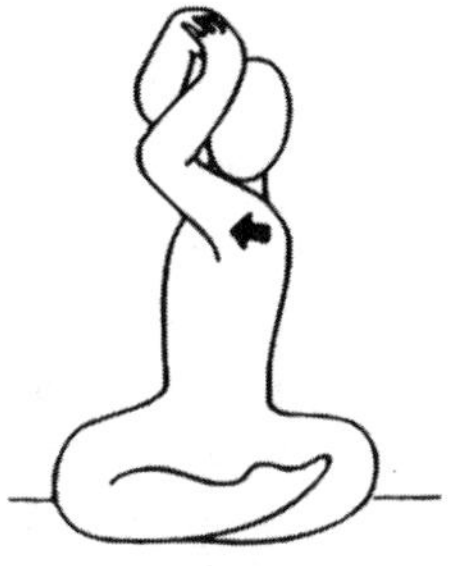

8c

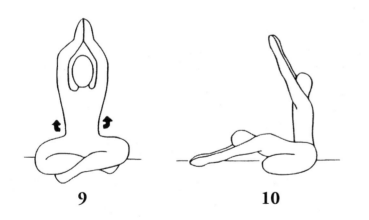

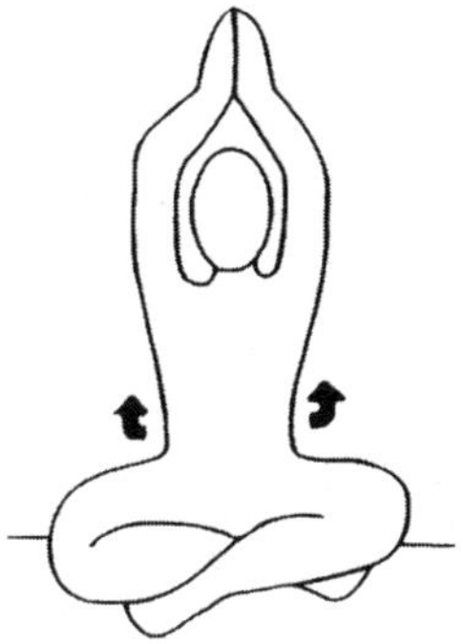

9

10

your face then return back to the sides. Release the mudra. Then begin the entire sequence again with the thumb and Mercury finger. It is important to bring the movement from behind the ear to the front of the forehead. You will circle around the horizontal center of the skull. 13 Minutes.

5. Make a wide V of your arms. Each arm is pointed up and out to the side at a 60° angle. The fingers of each hand are together but the thumb is stretched away from the hand. Your chin is tilted up and you breathe upward through the mouth. This is called the Akashic Breath. The breath is in rhythm with the music, "Sat Nam, Wahe Guru" (Indian version). The arms must not move. Breathe powerfully. 4 Minutes.
Inhale, tighten your arms and hands, and exhale. Hold your position and start to chant along with the mantra. Close your eyes and keep your face turned upward in this posture of ecstasy. 1 Minute. Inhale and relax. Shake out your shoulders.

Editor's Note: When this set was taught in 1986, the first drink was pure pineapple juice and the second drink was pure coconut juice. In 1993, Yogi Bhajan revised this to provide more vitamin C in each drink by mixing the two juices in the proportions given at the beginning of the set.

6. Arms are in front of the body and up at a 60 degree angle. The fingers are together with the palms flat, facing down. The tips of the thumbs touch each other. Close your eyes. Feel a ton of energy coming through your palms and pump your navel to the rhythm of "Bhor Na Marne Hoaa" by Ragi Sat Nam Singh. 9 Minutes. Inhale, stretch and as you hold your breath for 20 seconds, feel the life force energy in the third chakra.

7. Drink your second juice.

8. Lock your hands over your head in Venus lock. Twist your shoulders left and right. Your shoulders twist to the front of your body. This loosens up the rib cage and benefits the immune system. Sing along with "Sat Nam, Wahe Guru" (Indian version). 4 1/2 Minutes.

9. With your hands in Prayer Pose above your head, lock your thumbs and keep your arms as straight as possible. Twist left and right from the base of your spine. 5 Minutes. Yogi Bhajan played "Walking up the Mountain" by Krishna Kaur and Gurudass Singh during this and the following exercise.

10. Keep your arms in the same position and bend forward to touch the ground and rise back up. Bend at the area of the 3rd, 4th and 5th vertebrae, bend way down. 3 Minutes. Bend forward, rest your torso on the ground and stretch the lower back. 1-2 Minutes.

Balance of Prana and Apana

May 26, 1986

1

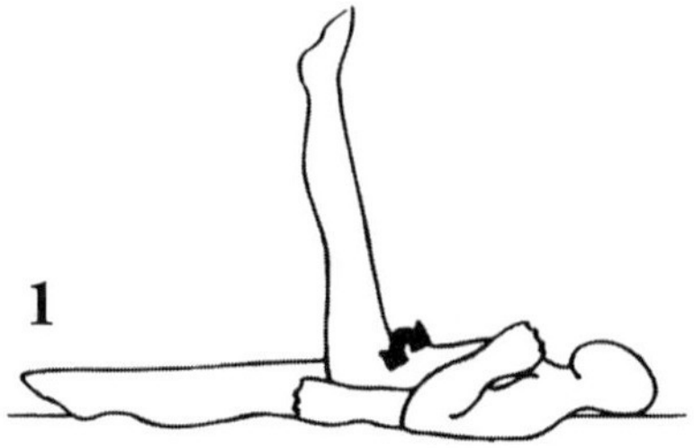

2a

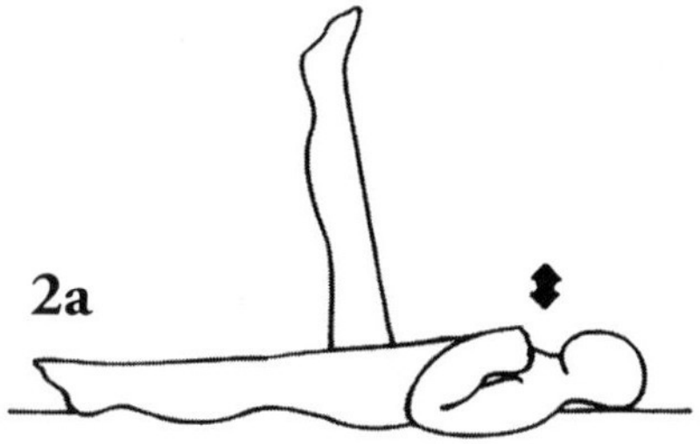

2b

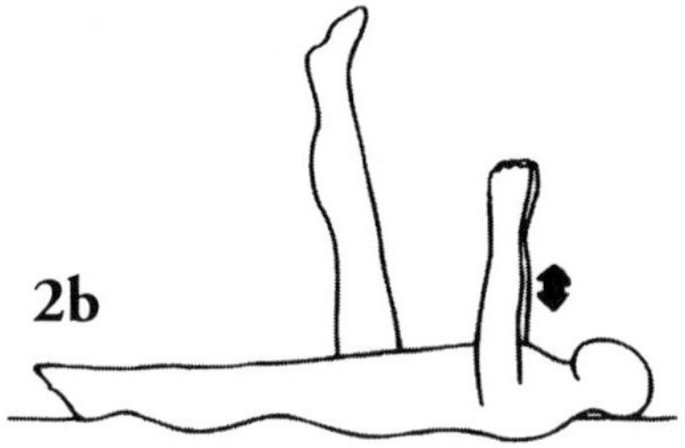

3

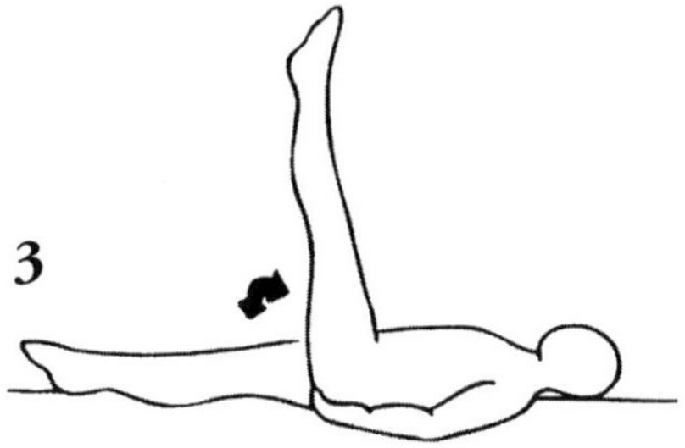

4

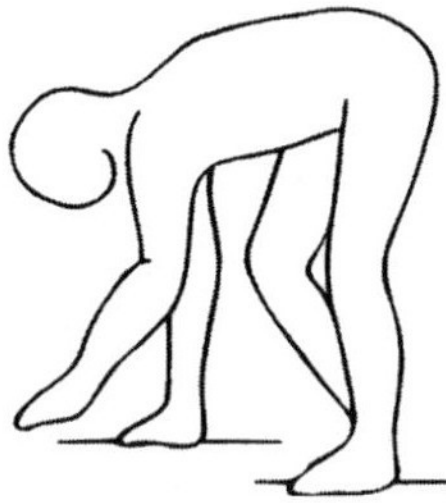

5a

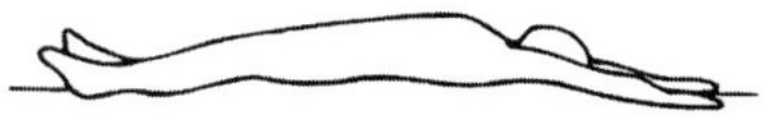

5b

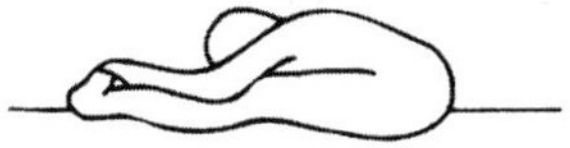

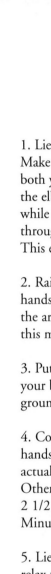

6

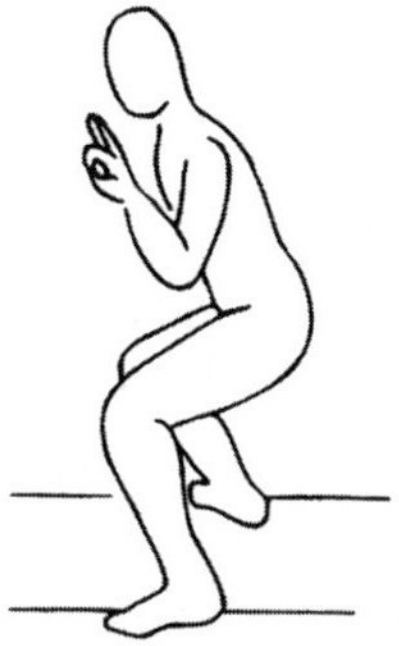

1. Lie down flat and raise your left leg to 90°. Rest your arms at your sides. Make fists of your hands. Feel that your fists are very heavy. Raise and lower both your hands at the same time as if you are lifting weights, bending at the elbows. Bring the fists to the shoulders and back down to the ground while keeping the upper arms on the ground. Your left leg stays up at 90° throughout the exercise. Move as fast as you can. 2 1/2 Minutes.
This exercise creates a balance between *prana* and *apana.*

2. Raise the right leg up to 90°. Raise both arms up to 90°. Keep your hands in relaxed fists. Bend the elbows and lower the arms and then raise the arms back up to 90°. Move the hands up and down together. Continue this motion as fast as you can. 1 Minute.

3. Put your hands under your buttocks with the palms up. (You are holding your buttocks in your hands) Do alternate leg lifts to 90° and back to the ground. 3 1/2 Minutes.

4. Come up on all fours, with your weight equally distributed on your hands and feet. Walk in one spot, but lift your arms and legs as if you were actually moving around. If you feel dizzy, you must stop this immediately. Otherwise, keep going and move fast. Your hips will move a lot.
2 1/2 - 3 Minutes. When you are super tense, do this exercise for 5 Minutes and you will be surprised how relaxed you will become.

5. Lie down flat, with the arms flat on the ground above your head, and relax your body. Rise up, bend forward, and touch your toes. Lie back down and continue. 108 times.

6. Stand up and bend your knees as if you were sitting in a chair. Keep your knees bent and your body as low as possible. Your elbows are bent and your hands are up at shoulder level with the thumb and forefinger in Gyan Mudra. Dance, staying in this position to the best of your ability. Play some rhythmic music (Yogi Bhajan played "Bhor Na Marne Hoaa" by Ragi Sat Nam Singh.) This exercise will give you youth and vigor. It will re-vibrate you. 10 Minutes. The same music is played throughout the remainder of the exercise set.

Much of the wisdom of the body's design is shown through the location and function of the subtle energies. ***Prana*** *is the energy of activity and inflow. Its central location is the lungs and heart.* ***Apana*** *is the energy of elimination and its central location is the area below the Navel Point and in the lower pelvis. This set creates a balanced and efficient flow between both areas and the subtle energies they hold. You will draw in energies you need and eliminate toxins, old thoughts, and sticky emotions.*

Gurucharan Singh

7

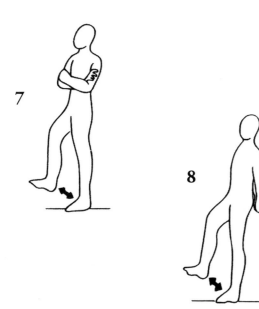

8

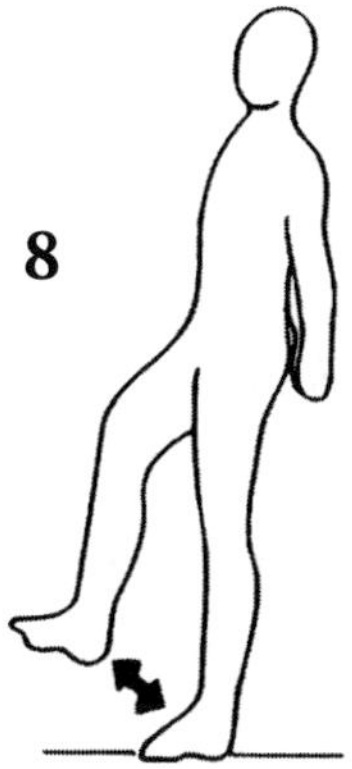

10

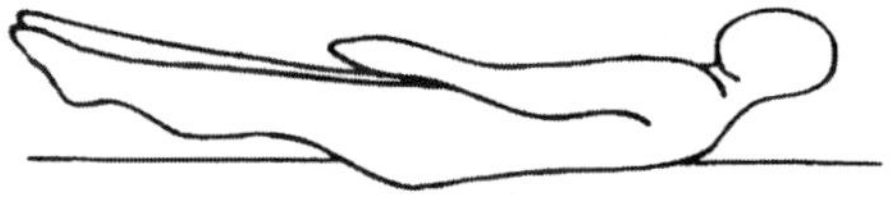

12a

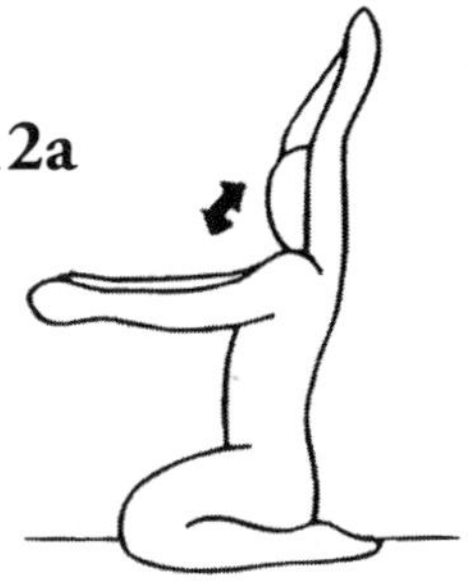

12b

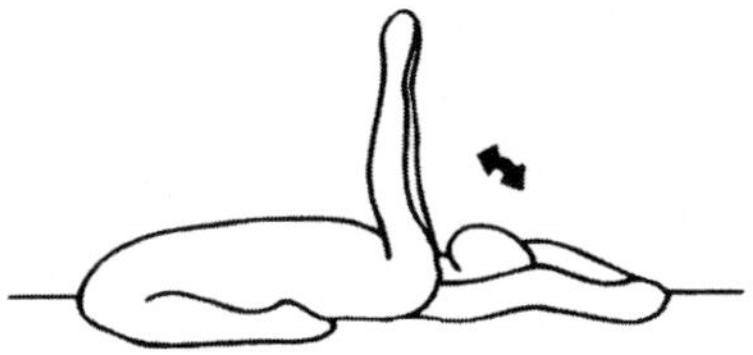

7. Straighten up and cross your arms over your chest. Kick out your feet alternately and continue to dance. 2 Minutes.

8. Lock your hands behind your back and continue to kick out your feet and dance. Kick hard! 2 Minutes.

9. Lie down flat on your back. Make fists of your hands and hammer your belly. Don't hit so hard that it hurts. Just hit hard enough to vigorously stimulate the belly area. Move fast! 2 Minutes.

10. Come up into Stretch Pose, but lift your legs up nine to twelve inches. The arms are straight with the fingers pointing toward the toes. The eyes are looking at the toes. Balance on the hip bone and let the navel vibrate. 1 Minute.

11. Stand up. Raise your arms, close your eyes, dance, and jump. Shake up the fat in your body. Move vigorously. 2 Minutes.

12. Sit on your heels and lock your hands together in front of your body. Your arms are out in front of your body parallel to the ground with the elbows straight but not locked. Raise your arms up to 90° and lower them back to the starting position as fast as you can. 1 Minute. Continue this movement in the same posture, while slowly and gradually lowering yourself onto your back. Keep moving the arms. 1/2 Minute. Rise up again while still moving the arms. Relax.

13. Come sitting in Easy Pose with your hands in Gyan Mudra. Meditate and try not to listen to the music. Concentrate not to listen. After 5 Minutes of this, begin to sing along with the music. 4 Minutes. Deeply inhale and exhale a total of three times to finish.

Chakras, Physical Wisdom and Healing

By Gurucharan Singh Khalsa, PhD, Director of Training

Part of the physical wisdom we find in the body comes from its connection to a subtle realm. The body is physical. We can see it with our eyes. But the body also has another field of energy and activity that we cannot see with the eye. Yogis who have trained themselves to see this energy field say it is like light radiating in complex patterns from each cell of the body. It is fluid and constantly moving. In that whirlpool of activity, there are subtle vortexes that interconnect the subtle and physical realms. These centers of transformation and connection are called chakras. These chakras interact with and influence our thoughts, moods, health, and other bodily functions. They exchange energy bi-directionally—from gross to subtle and from subtle to gross. They are doorways of consciousness.

There are eight major chakras. While they are associated with areas of the body, in actuality, they shift around like swirls in water. When the mind and body are healthy and vital, they tend to project through specific areas. The First Chakra is near the base of the spine and anus. The Second Chakra is near the sex organs and the 3rd and 4th vertebrae. The Third Chakra is near the Navel Point. The Fourth Chakra is near the Heart Center and is associated with the thymus gland. The Fifth Chakra is near the throat and is associated with the thyroid gland. The Sixth Chakra is near the top of the nose, associated with the pituitary gland. The Seventh Chakra is near the crown of the head, associated with the pineal gland.

The Eighth Chakra is the circumvent field that surrounds the entire body. It is like a filter and shield which encloses the other chakras. There are hundreds of other smaller chakras attached to other organs and to meridian points, but they are commanded through this central system. All the main chakras are connected by a channel of energy called the Shushmuna that travels up the center of the spine and around the brain.

The following meditations strengthen and tune each chakra as well as interconnect them into a fully functional system. Practicing these meditations can contribute to the healing of many illnesses—mental, emotional, and physical. You can practice them in any order. Each technique is complete and balanced in itself. It will open, adjust, and strengthen the chakra. You can have a great benefit from practicing any one of them for just one session or you may decide to do a meditation for one particular chakra for 40 days. The last meditation, Sodarshan Chakra Kriya, is a most beautiful technique. It balances the flow of energy through all the chakras so you make good decisions and attract appropriate resources to your purposes.

Kundalini Yoga opens, maintains, and develops the chakra system in the subtle body. It is the fastest and most potent approach discovered by the ancient sages. These techniques were closely guarded secrets. Yogi Bhajan, under the blessing of Guru Ram Das, has made all these techniques openly available without restriction. He said, "The Age of Aquarius is dawning and every person has the opportunity to elevate themselves through sadhana, techniques, and commitment. The old ways will quickly change in this fast, electronic age of light. I am just a postman for those souls that have earned the destiny to elevate themselves."

Meditation for the First Chakra

January 22 & 23, 1991

Posture: Sit in a comfortable position such as Easy Pose, making sure that your spine is straight.

Starting Position: Your arms are held out to your sides with the elbows bent and the palms of your hands facing each other. The palms are angled towards each other at a 60° angle. (To put the hands in the correct position, begin by holding them with the palms facing downward. Tilt the inner edge of each hand up 60° so that the thumbs and forefingers are the highest part of the tilted plane of the hand.)

In Kundalini Yoga we don't initiate anybody. A person has to initiate himself or herself and learn the discipline.

Yogi Bhajan

Warm Up: The initial warm-up involves moving your hands slowly toward each other from the starting position, simultaneously squeezing the anus until the hands meet at the center of your body at which time the contraction of the anus is released. Practicing this for a few Minutes will give you the feel of the meditation before all the other elements are added.

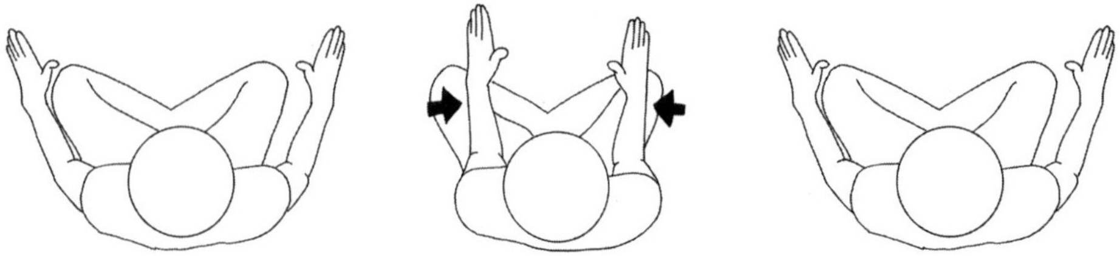

Mantra: The meditation is done to Nirinjan Kaur and Guru Prem Singh's version of "Hummee Hum, Brahm Hum." The chanting is performed in a special way: Your tongue is recessed; that is, it is relaxed and flat in the bottom of your mouth and is not used to chant the mantra. This will produce a pressure that will be felt in the cheekbone area.

Focus: The eyes are focused at the tip of the nose.

Meditation: From the starting position, with a straight spine and eyes focused at the tip of the nose, the hands are brought together at the center of the body (similar to clapping) in two distinct and strong moves. The first move brings the hands half-way in as you chant "Hummee Hum" with the recessed tongue. The hands stop briefly and begin to move again as you chant "Brahm Hum" bringing the hands together in front of the body. When the hands move, you squeeze the anus and maintain that contraction until the hands touch and then you relax the anus, return your hands to the starting position and begin again.

Time: Begin with 11 Minutes and slowly work up to 31 Minutes.

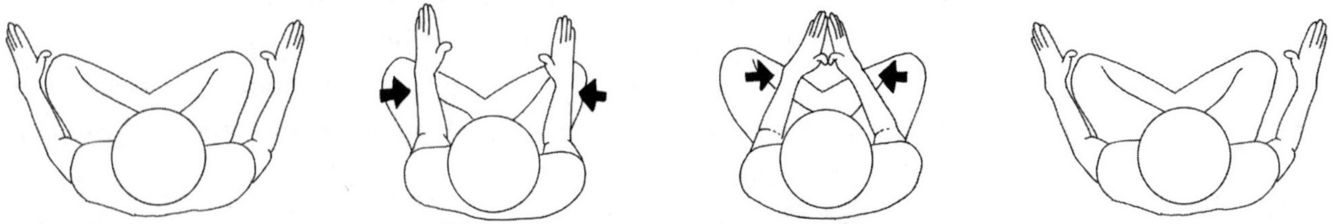

Meditation for the Second Chakra

January 29 & 30, 1991

Posture: Sit in a comfortable sitting position such as Easy Pose, making sure that your spine is straight.

Starting Position: Your arms are out to the sides, elbows bent with the palms of the hands facing each other about shoulder width apart. The palms are angled in toward each other at a 60° angle. (To put the hands in the correct position, begin by holding them with the palms facing downward. Tilt the inner edge of each hand up 60° so that the thumbs and forefingers are the highest part of the tilted plane of the hand.)

Mantra: The meditation is done to Nirinjan Kaur and Guru Prem Singh's version of "Ek Ong Kar, Sat Gur Prasad." There is no chanting but the movement of the meditation is done with the rhythm of the music.

Focus: The eyes are focused at the tip of the nose.

If there is a purpose other than compassion in the relationships in your life, you will also find pain in those relationships.

Yogi Bhajan

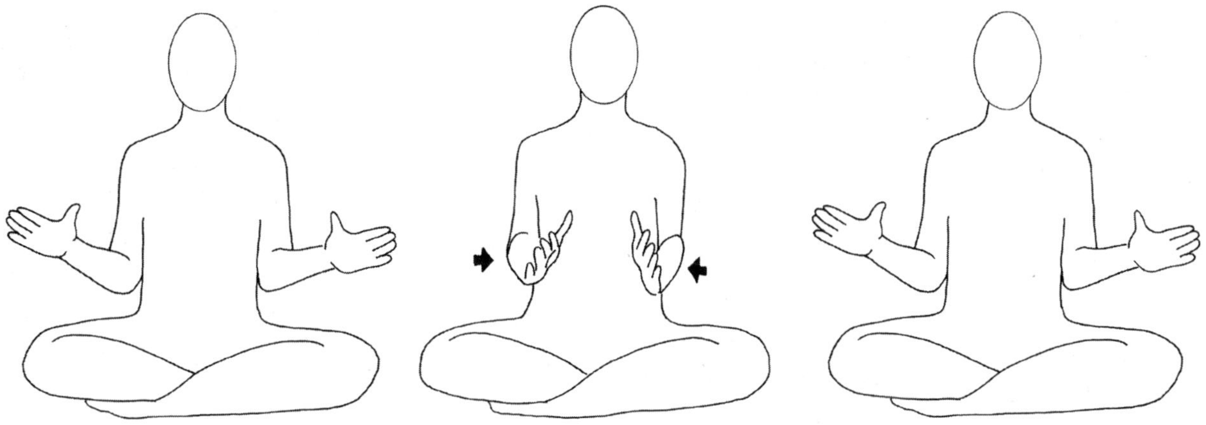

Meditation: From the starting position, bring the hands towards each other at the center of the body, but do not let them touch. This movement is strong and sharp, something like a clap without touching the hands. As the hands move inward, tighten the sex organ and release it as the hands move back to the starting position. For men the tightening is centered at the base of the sex organ and for women, the contraction includes the clitoris. This is not a mul bhand, the anus and Navel Point are not contracted with the sex organ.

Time: Begin with 11 Minutes and slowly work up to 31 Minutes.

To Finish: Inhale and hold the breath and tighten and tense every muscle in the body. Hold for 15 seconds and then relax. Repeat the sequence: inhaling, holding the breath, tensing the body, and exhaling 2 more times.

Meditation for the Third Chakra

February 5 & 6, 1991

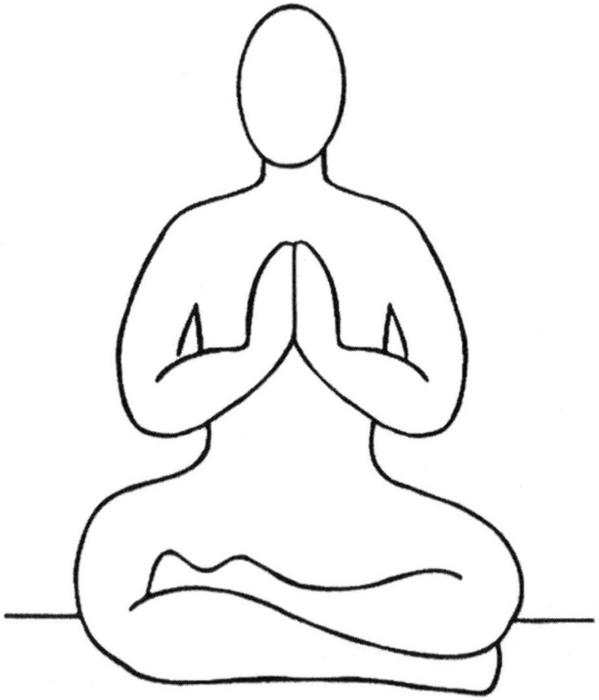

Posture: Sit in Easy Pose, making sure that your spine is straight.

Starting Position: The elbows are bent and the hands are in Prayer Pose. All parts of the palms are touching and pressing together with equal force.

Mantra: The meditation is done to Nirinjan Kaur and Guru Prem Singh's version of "Humee Hum, Brahm Hum." The chanting is done with the tip of the tongue.

You need grit. You need nervous strength. You need the totality of you.

Yogi Bhajan

Focus: The eyes are focused at the tip of the nose.

Meditation: Chant "Humee" with the tip of the tongue and press the hands together as you pull the Navel Point in and then release it. Chant "Hum" again with the tip of the tongue as you press the hands together and pull in on the navel and release. Chant "Brahm" and again apply the pressure on the hands and the pull on the navel and release. Chant "Hum" and again repeat the pressure, the pull, and the release.

(Yogi Bhajan said that the hand press was a compression, like the beat of the heart.)

Time: Do this meditation only for 11 Minutes.

To Finish: Inhale and hold the breath, pull in on the navel and press the tip of the tongue against the roof of the mouth. Hold for 15 seconds and exhale. Repeat the sequence: inhaling, holding the breath, pulling in on the navel, pressing the tip of the tongue against the roof of the mouth and exhaling 2 more times. Relax.

When this meditation has been perfected in this form, it may be practiced with the Root Lock applied.

Meditation for the Fourth Chakra I

February 12, 1991

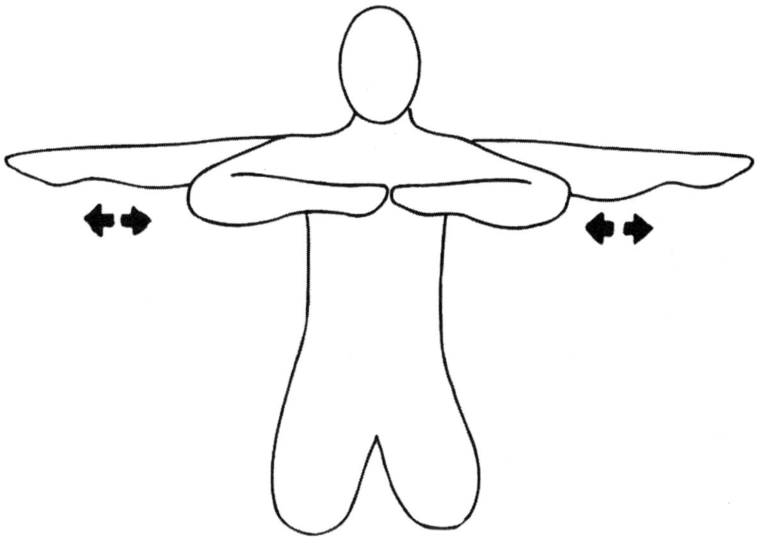

Posture: Sit on your heels with a straight spine.

Position: The upper arms are parallel to the ground, on the same level as the shoulders. The elbows are bent and the fingertips are nearly touching each other at the center of the chest near the Heart Center. The hands are flat with the palms facing downward.

Trust is the fiber of love.

Yogi Bhajan

Mantra: The meditation is done to the rhythm of "Humee Hum, Brahm Hum" by Nirinjan Kaur and Guru Prem Singh. The meditation is silent, you do not chant along with the mantra.

Focus: The eyes are focused at the tip of the nose.

Meditation: From the starting position, the hands and forearms move out to the sides palms facing down. Pull the Navel Point in strongly and lift the solar plexus and diaphragm slightly in a focused motion. As the arms move back in, the navel is released. The navel is pulled in as the arms again move back out to the sides. Continue this movement using the rhythm of the music to set the pace.

Time: 11 Minutes.

To Finish: Inhale and hold the breath 15 seconds and release. Repeat this two more times and relax.

Meditation for the Fourth Chakra II

February 13, 1991

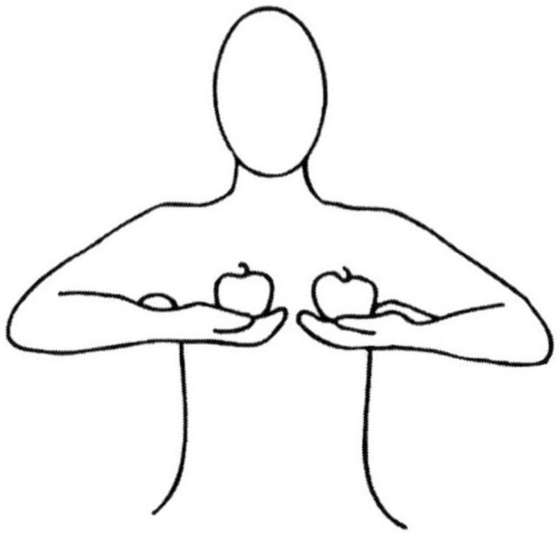

Mudra for 2

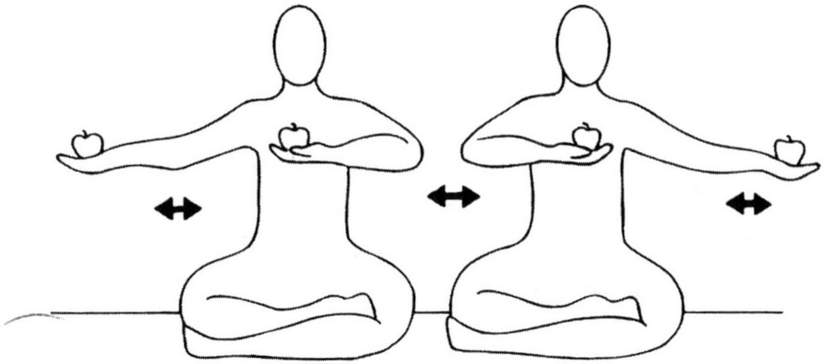

You will need two apples for this kriya.

Posture: Sit in Easy Pose with a straight spine.

Position: This meditation is done holding an apple in the palm of each hand. Your elbows are bent with your forearms parallel to the ground. The hands are palms up and the fingertips are nearly touching each other at the center of the chest, near your Heart Center. Each hand is relaxed and holds the apple without gripping it.

Mantra: Chant along with Nirinjan Kaur and Guru Prem Singh's "Humee Hum, Brahm Hum" using the tip of the tongue when you chant.

Focus: The eyes are focused at the tip of the nose.

Meditation: From the starting position, the hands move in and out alternately. As one hand brings an apple in and offers it to your Heart Center, the other hand moves out to the side and offers its apple to the Universe.

Note: This meditation is to be done only in the morning between 6 am and 9 am. It may be practiced for 11 Minutes.

To Finish: Inhale, hold the breath 15 seconds, and release. Repeat this two more times and relax. You may now eat your apples

After three Minutes of this exercise, you will experience yourself becoming cranky and serious. If you can smile at this time it will open your Heart Center.

Yogi Bhajan

Meditation for the Fifth Chakra

February 19 & 20, 1991

Posture: Sit in Easy Pose, with a straight spine.

Position: Thumb and forefinger are in Gyan Mudra, the other fingers are relaxed and slightly curved. The hands are on the knees. The neck is absolutely straight with the chin pulled in. This is Jalandhar Bandh or Neck Lock. The chest is lifted and the chin rests in the notch between the collar bones at the top of the breast bone. The head stays level without tilting forward. The spine in the neck is straight. The chin is pulled in, the chest is out and there is little weight on the buttocks. Yogi Bhajan mentioned that when the Neck Lock is properly applied, a stretch can be felt in the deltoid muscles.

Mantra: The meditation is done to Nirinjan Kaur and Guru Prem Singh's version of "Humee Hum, Brahm Hum." The chanting is done with the root of the tongue, the pressure is felt in the throat.

Focus: The eyes are focused at the tip of the nose.

Meditation: In Jalandhar Bandh, chant the mantra with the root of the tongue.

Time: 11 Minutes.

Benefits: Practicing this kriya for 11 Minutes a day for 18 months will keep you young in spirit and looks.

Those who do not know how to live to their words shall never have the knowledge to know God.

Yogi Bhajan

Meditation for the Sixth Chakra

March 5, 1991

The Sixth Chakra is located where the root of the nose reaches the skull. This chakra, the pituitary gland, controls the entire glandular system.

Posture: Sit in Easy Pose, with a straight spine.

Meditation: Look at the tip of your nose (the "lotus tip") for 11 Minutes a day between the hours of 4 am and 8 am local time and you shall control the entire glandular system for the next 24 hours and the chemistry of the blood will change for the better.

Patience gives you the power to practice; practice gives you power that leads you to perfection.

Yogi Bhajan

Meditation for the Seventh and Eighth Chakras

Posture: Sit in Easy Pose with the spine straight. Hands are in Gyan Mudra.

Focus: Eyes are focused on the tip of the nose.

Meditation: Chant "Ang Sang Wahe Guru" for 31 Minutes.

To Finish: Inhale deeply and hold the breath as long as possible. Exhale. Repeat two more times.

This meditation exalts the intuition.

Gurucharan Singh

Sodarshan Chakra Kriya

August 1991 and December 12, 1990

Posture: Sit with a straight spine.

Focus: The eyes are focused at the tip of the nose.

Meditation: Block off the right nostril with the right thumb. Inhale slowly and deeply through the left nostril. Hold the breath. Mentally chant "Wahe Guru" sixteen times, pumping the Navel Point once on "Wha", once on "Hey", and once on "Guru". (You pump the navel three times with each complete repetition of "Wahe Guru" and you chant "Wahe Guru" sixteen times. Therefore on each breath, you pump the Navel Point 48 times.) Unblock the right nostril. Use the right index finger (little finger may also be used) to block off the left nostril and exhale slowly and completely through the right nostril. Continue.

Time: 31 or 62 Minutes a day. There is no time, no place, no space, and no condition attached to this mantra.

If you are going to clean your own subconscious garbage, you must estimate and clean it as fast as you can or as slow as you want. You have to decide how much time you have to clean up your garbage pit. So, start with 31 Minutes, then after a while do it for 40 Minutes, and then for 62 Minutes. Take time to graduate in it.

If you can do this meditation for 62 Minutes to start with and develop it to the point that you can do it for 2 1/2 hours a day, it makes out of you a perfect superbeing. It purifies, takes care of the human life and makes a human perfect, saintly, successful, and qualified. This meditation also gives one the pranic power. This kriya never fails. It can give one all the inner happiness and bring one to a state of ecstasy in life.

To Finish: Inhale, hold 5-10 seconds, exhale. Then stretch and shake every part of your body for about 1 Minute so that the energy may spread.

Of all the 20 types of yoga, including Kundalini Yoga, this is the highest kriya. This meditation cuts through all darkness. The name, Sodarshan Chakra Kriya, means the Kriya for Perfect Purification of the Chakras. It will give you a new start. It is the simplest kriya, but at the same time the hardest. It cuts through all barriers of the neurotic or psychotic inside nature. When a person is in a very bad state, techniques imposed from the outside will not work. The pressure has to be stimulated from within. The tragedy of life is when the subconscious releases garbage into the conscious mind. This kriya invokes the Kundalini energy to give you the necessary vitality and intuition to combat the negative effects of the unchanneled subconscious mind.

Yogi Bhajan

More Kundalini Meditations for Physical Wisdom

By Gurucharan Singh Khalsa, PhD, Director of Training

This collection of meditations will further enhance the use of your physical wisdom. They are practical techniques that fight stress, enhance intuition, and increase basic life energy. Yogi Bhajan has shared literally hundreds of meditation techniques. These meditations directly expand your life, coping with challenge, and experiencing your physical wisdom.

Meditation is the mindful direction of your awareness. It can be active, passive, ecstatic, serious, quiet, loud, in retreat, or during daily activities. Not all meditations do the same thing. It is like climbing a mountain. All paths lead to the top, but some paths develop leg strength (straight up the north wall), some develop aesthetic sense (the gradual path along the fields of flowers), and some enhance interpersonal skills (the path that crosses all the way stations and camps). All meditations will develop self-mastery and will engage aspects of the mind so you can live from your soul and awareness. Each meditation has its own signature and distinct effects. That is the power and vastness of Kundalini Yoga in the Raja Yoga tradition of Guru Ram Das. There are entire schools of practice based on one or two meditations. Kundalini is the compilation of effective meditations from all authentic endeavors across many times and cultures. Its diversity is both challenging and useful. Any person can find a meditation that fits his or her own need, level of accomplishment, temperament, and goals.

Adjust the Brain and Increase Intelligence

March 25, 1992

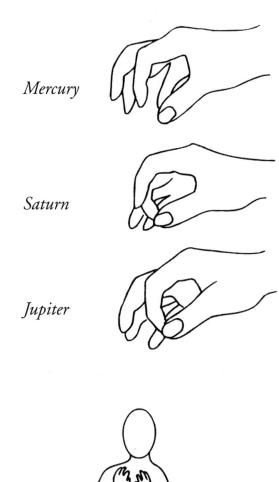

Mercury

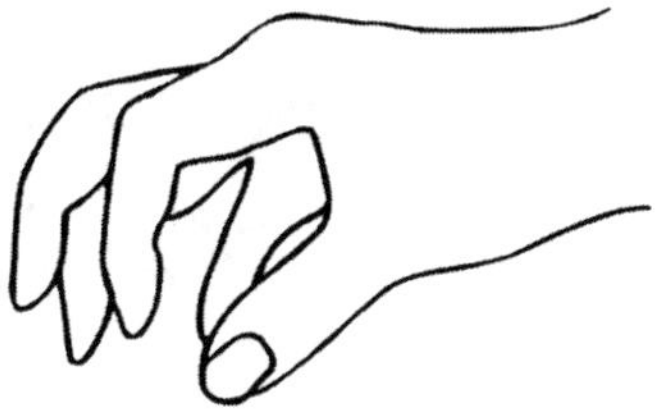

Saturn

Jupiter

Sit in Easy Pose and do this mudra with both hands at the same time. First touch the thumb and pinkie (Mercury finger), then touch the thumb and middle (Saturn) finger, and then touch the thumb and index (Jupiter) finger. Continue this sequence but do not touch the thumb and ring (Sun) finger.

Keeping your legs in Easy Pose, lift and release both knees at the same time as you touch each finger with the thumb. Legs move up and down like a butterfly flapping its wings. Keep the arms bent near the torso, palms toward the body as you play the fingertips and lift the knees.

Chant "Humee Hum, Brahm Hum" using Nirinjan Kaur's version of the mantra. Chant touching the tip of the tongue to the upper palate. When properly chanted in this manner, it will sound strange. One word of the mantra corresponds with one touch of finger and thumb.

Focus: Eyes are focused at the tip of the nose.

Time: 31 Minutes

This meditation can be taught to children in either their third or fourth year. The practice time can be adjusted to suit their attention span.

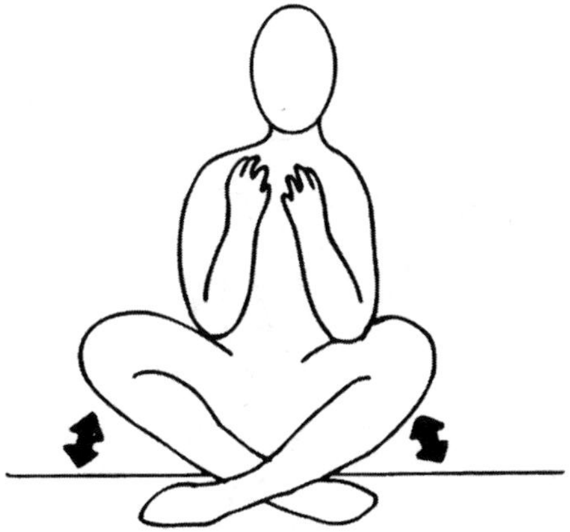

1

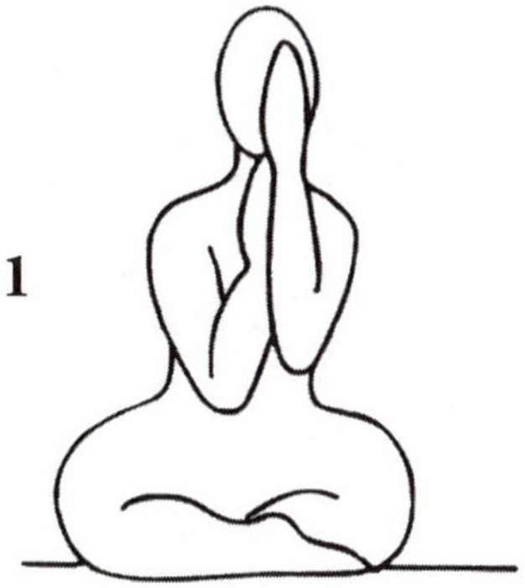

2

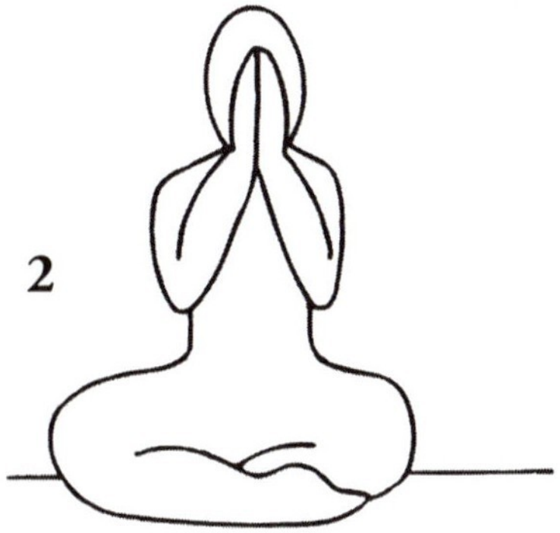

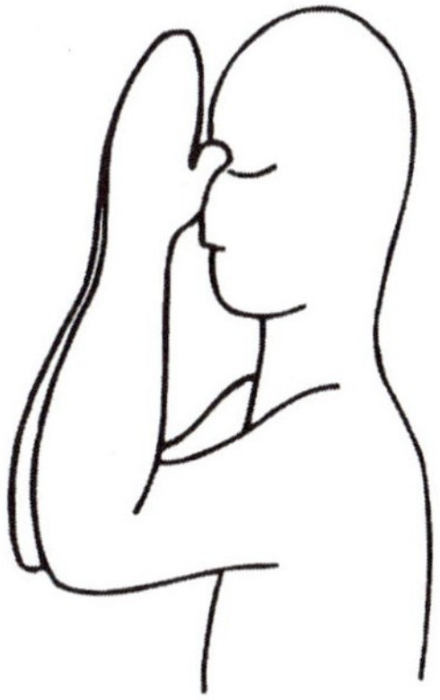

2
Side view

3

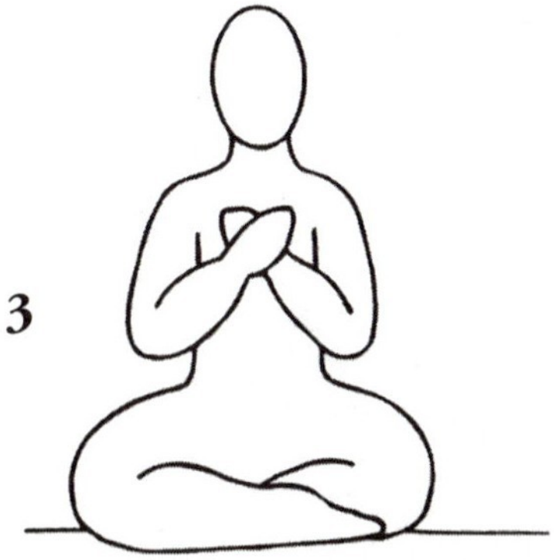

Inner Assessment

Summer 1992

1. **To Know Your Inner Balance:**
Sit in Easy Pose, with your eyes closed, focusing at the third eye point. Bring the hands into Prayer Pose at the center of the chest. Slide the left hand upward until it is higher than the right, with the left palm facing to the right side. The right palm faces left and touches the left arm just below the wrist. Breathe as long and slowly as you can. 3-11 Minutes.

2. **To Know Your Inner Projection:**
Sit in Easy Pose with the eyes closed, focusing at the third eye point. Your thumbs are hooked into the hollows on either side of the bridge of your nose. Slowly close the palms into Prayer Pose, closing from the bottom of the side of the palms upward, touching the sides of the fingers last. Hold this position. Breathe as long and slowly as you can. 3-11 Minutes.

3. **To Know Your Inner Strength:**
Sit in Easy Pose with the eyes closed, focusing at the third eye point. Breathe as long and slowly as you can. Place your right hand over your left at your Heart Center and press as hard as you can, maintaining the pressure throughout the meditation. 3-11 Minutes.

See God in all. See opportunity in all. See grace in all. With that impact, walk your life very gracefully.

Yogi Bhajan

Transition into the Aquarian Age

December 1, 1993

For those born in the Piscean Age, the transition into the Aquarian Age will create difficulties. Those of us who have been born in the old age will be living in an era when the old ways will not work. As we move deeper into the 21-year cusp period of the new age (from November 1991 to November 2012) there will be a feeling of emptiness inside that will increase every year. This meditation will help to minimize the effects of this process.

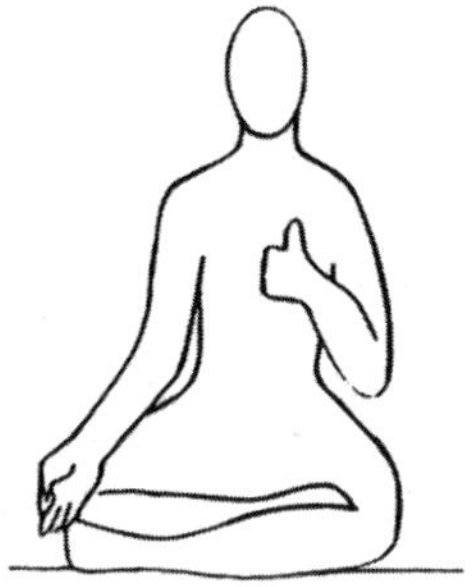

1

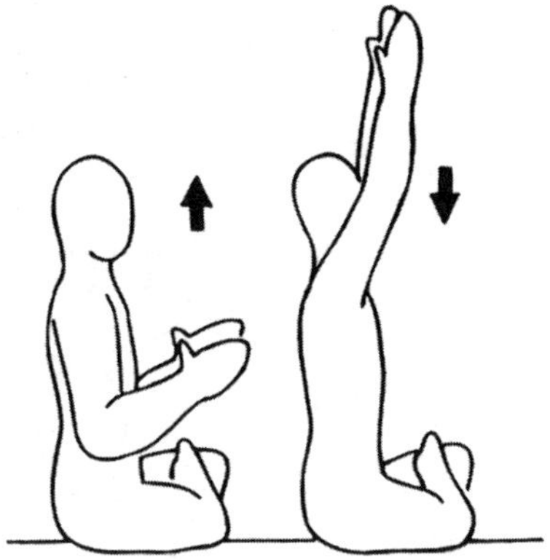

2

1. Sit in Easy Pose with your left elbow bent comfortably at your side and your left hand in front of your Heart Center. Your left hand is in a fist with the thumb pointing either straight up or bent backward. (Some people can bend their thumbs backward, and others can't. Do it whichever way is natural for you.) Your right hand is in Gyan Mudra and resting on your right knee. Inhale slowly, hold, and slowly exhale so that you breathe exactly 3 times per minute. Continue for 11 Minutes. You can time yourself by watching the second hand of a clock, by mentally counting off the 20 second segments, or by using the thumb of your right hand to mark time by touching each of the three segments of your fingers up to 20 touches.

2. Bring both elbows to the sides of your chest with your palms facing each other and the fingers pointing straight forward. Inhale and, while holding the breath, raise your hands up over your head and bring them back down to your sides 8 times. Then exhale. Stretch up and come down strongly and quickly. Do this cycle 5 times.

3a
Starting position

3b
Circling outward

3c
To this point

3. Still sitting in Easy Pose, point the Jupiter (index) finger of each hand straight out while curling the remaining three fingers into a fist. Secure the Saturn (middle) finger with the thumb. Move your hands out to the sides while rotating your hands to the outside in small circles. When your arms are fully extended, move your hands back to your sides in a straight line while rotating your hands to the inside in small circles. Continue for 5 Minutes.

4. To finish: inhale, hold your breath, squeeze your body tightly, and exhale. Repeat this 2 more times.

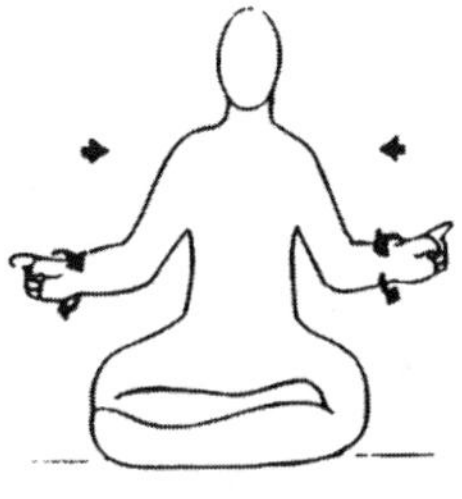

3d
Circling inward

3e
Back to the starting position

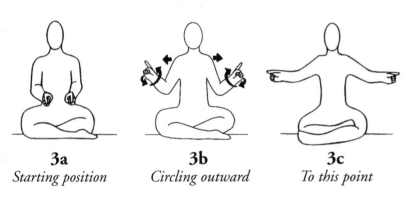

Meditation for the Navel Center, Heart Center, Throat Center and Third Eye

Spring 1992

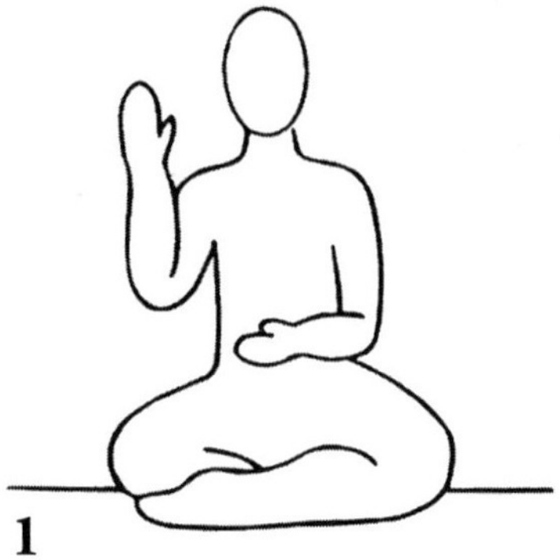

1

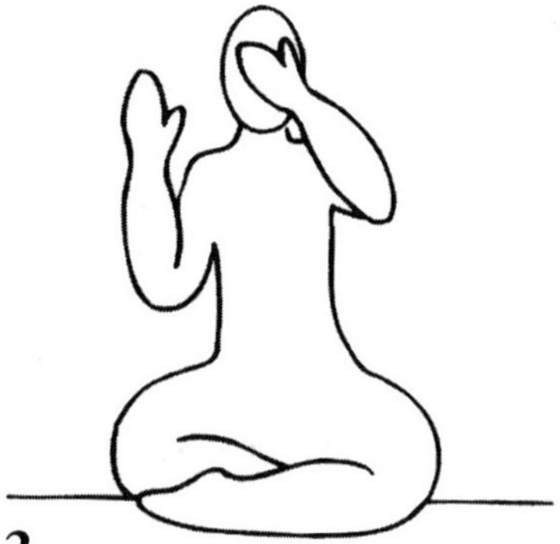

2

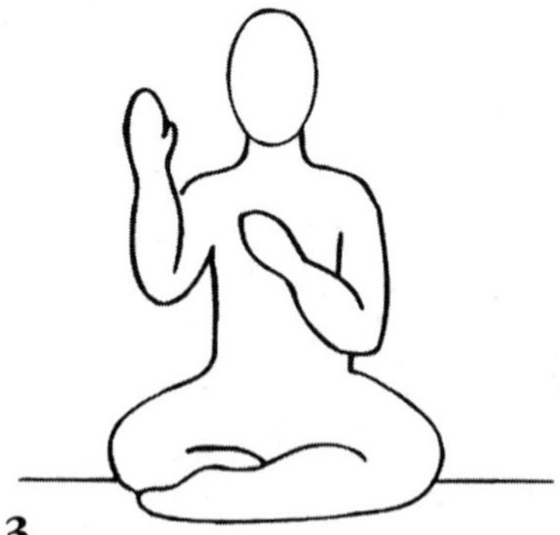

3

1. Sit in Easy Pose. Put the center of your left palm over your Navel Point and bend your right arm so that the forearm is at 90°. The palm is flat and facing forward. The fingers point straight up. Look at the tip of your nose and chant "Har Singh, Nar Singh, Neel Narayan" with Nirinjan Kaur's version of the mantra. Chant with the tip of your tongue. 3 Minutes.

2. Put your left palm on your forehead and keep the right arm as in position 1. Look at the tip of your nose and chant "Sat Siri, Siri Akal" with Nirinjan Kaur's version of the mantra. Chant with the tip of your tongue. 3 Minutes.

3. Repeat Exercise 1 for 1 1/2 Minutes.

4. Put your left palm on your Heart Center. Keep your right arm the same as in the previous exercises. Look at the tip of your nose and chant "Har Nar Wahe Guru" using the version by Nirinjan Kaur. Chant with the tip of your tongue. 1 Minute.

Relax.

If the tip of your tongue touches the upper palate while you chant, it stimulates 84 meridian points. This gives you the power and energy to win.

Yogi Bhajan

To Know Through Intuition

March 10, 1993

1

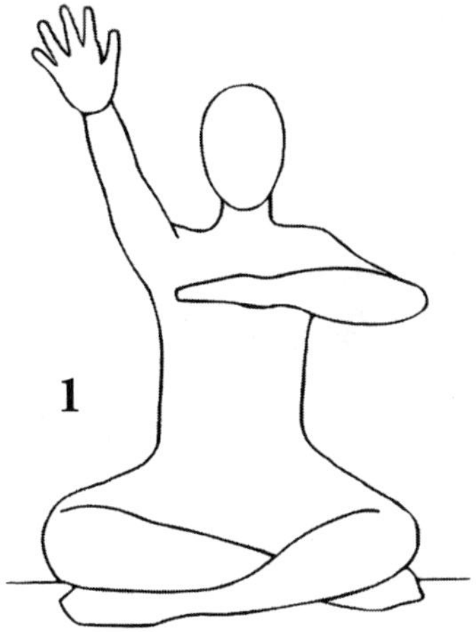

2

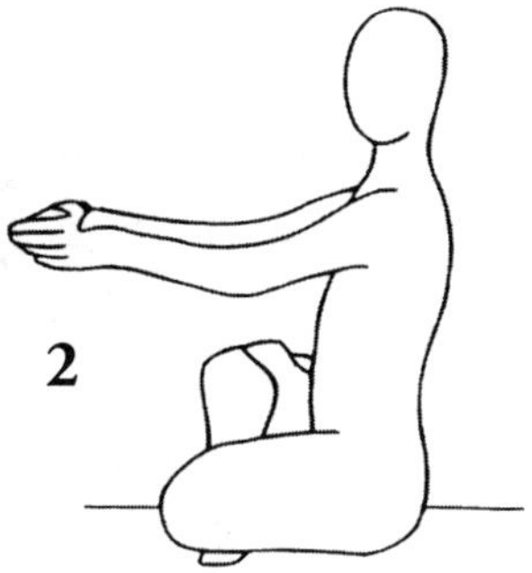

3

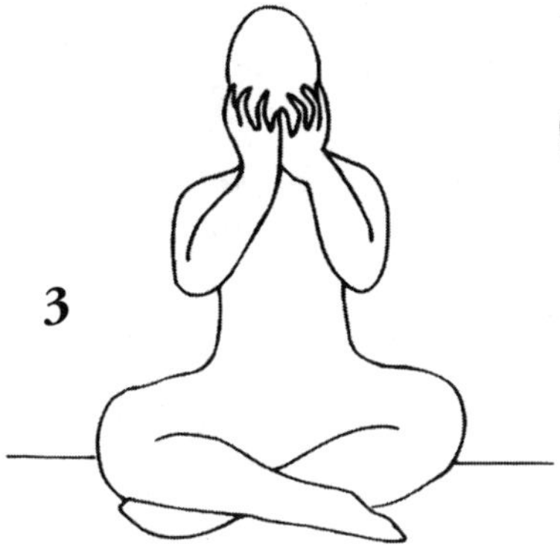

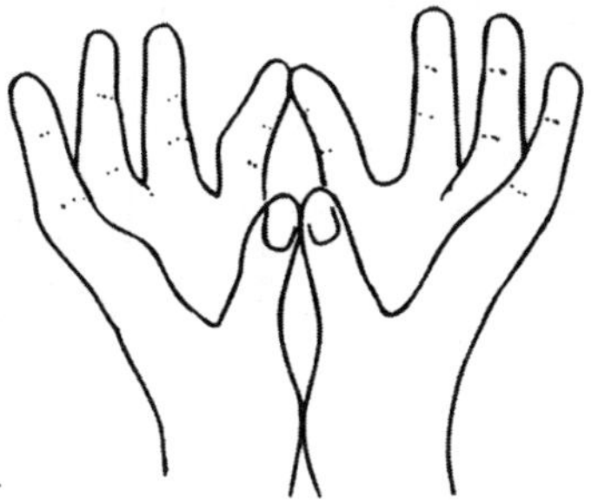

Lotus mudra for exercise 3

4

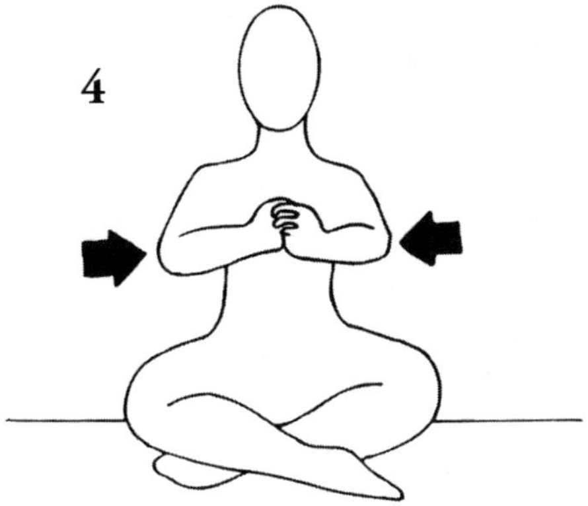

1. Sit in Easy Pose. The left elbow is bent, the hand is in front of the Heart Center, and the palm is flat and faces the floor. The right arm is extended out to the front at a 60° angle. Close your eyes and breathe slowly and honestly. (Work up to breathing only one breath per minute). Feel the Divine Presence around you. 11 Minutes.

To finish: Stay in the posture, inhale deep, hold the breath 10 seconds as you tighten all the muscles of the body, and exhale. Repeat 2 more times. Relax, roll your shoulders, stretch your arms and rib cage.

2. In Easy Pose, your arms are extended straight out in front of your chest with the palms touching and the thumbs locked over each other. Close your eyes and whistle a song of your choice. 7 Minutes. This posture affects the parathyroid and you may feel a pressure in your neck.

3. Still in Easy Pose, put your hands in a Lotus Mudra about at eye level. Relax the entire body but hold the hand position strongly. Close your eyes for 3 Minutes. This is an intertwined action when one part of the body in a confined posture becomes the antenna and the rest of the body is relaxed to receive.

4. Inhale and clasp your hands in front of your Heart Center and press as hard as you can. Exhale and repeat 2 more times. Then relax, talk, and ground yourself for a few moments.

Meditation and life are very interlocked. It is important to be able to know what is going on beneath the surface of situations. Ordinarily untrained people can do this 15% of the time, but the ideal is to have your intuition work at the 60% level or higher. This meditation builds your intuitive capacity.

Eliminate Tension and Stress

March 9,1993

1

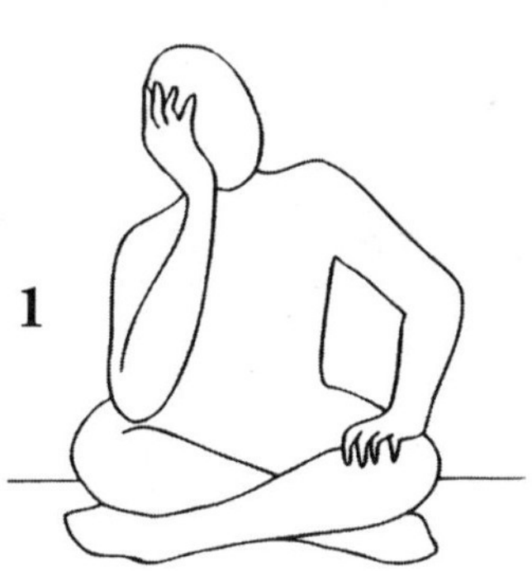

1. **Relaxing Buddha:** a relaxing pose that will release tension and stress in just 11 Minutes. Sit in Easy Pose. Your right elbow is bent and resting on the right knee. Lean your right cheekbone on the palm of your right hand with the fingers loosely covering the right half of your forehead. Close your eyes and just relax. This pose will put pressure on your liver, so just relax and let the body adjust to it. If you want to really relax, play the "Guru Ram Das Lullaby" as you do this meditation. 11 Minutes.

A most powerful combination against stress is to do the Relaxing Buddha meditation and then do 31 Minutes of breathing only one breath per minute (inhale 20 seconds, hold 20 seconds, and exhale 20 seconds). It will bring you to a state of calmness that will win the game of life.

Yogi Bhajan

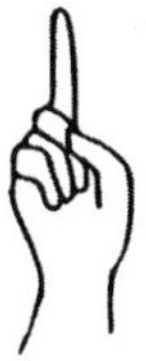

right hand position

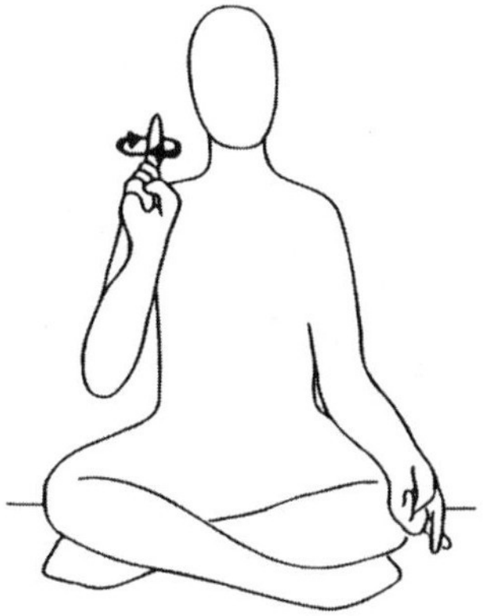

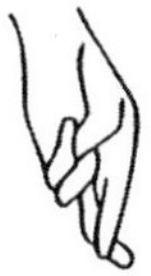

left hand position

2

2. **To Experience the Jupiter Energy:**
Sit in Easy Pose. Left hand mudra: the Saturn (middle) finger crosses over the back of the Jupiter (index) finger. The other two fingers are closed and locked down with the thumb. The back of the left hand rests on the left knee.

Right hand mudra: the Jupiter (index) finger extends straight up and the other fingers are closed and locked down with the thumb. The right elbow is bent and the right hand is about chin level. Close your eyes, relax, and quickly move the Jupiter finger around in a circle. Only the Jupiter finger moves.

Concentrate on moving the Jupiter finger. Listen to "Ang Sang Wahe Guru" by Nirinjan Kaur. 11 Minutes. To finish: inhale, keep the finger moving, and tighten all the muscles of the body as you hold the breath for 10 seconds. Exhale and repeat two more times.

This meditation can release tension and call in the Jupiter energy of prosperity and expansion.

3

3. **To Get Rid of Tension so You Can Live:**
To let it all go. Sit in Easy Pose. Extend your arms out and down with the palms up. Circle your extended arms inward and upward and continue around to complete the circle. Really push hard as you move upward.
3 Minutes. Then inhale deeply and relax.

Normally there is so much tension in life that we are all numb. We miss opportunities through a lack of sensitivity.

Yogi Bhajan

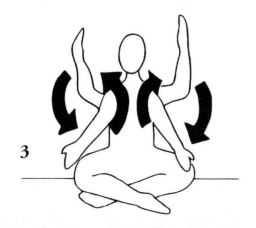

Techniques to Fight Fatigue

March 1992

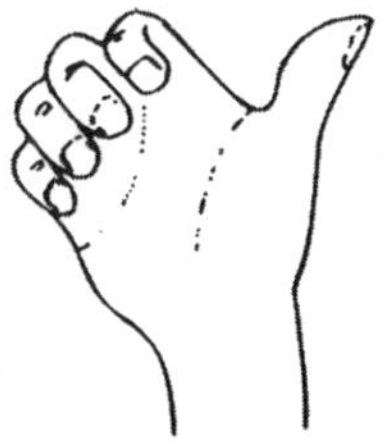

Mudra for exercise 1

1

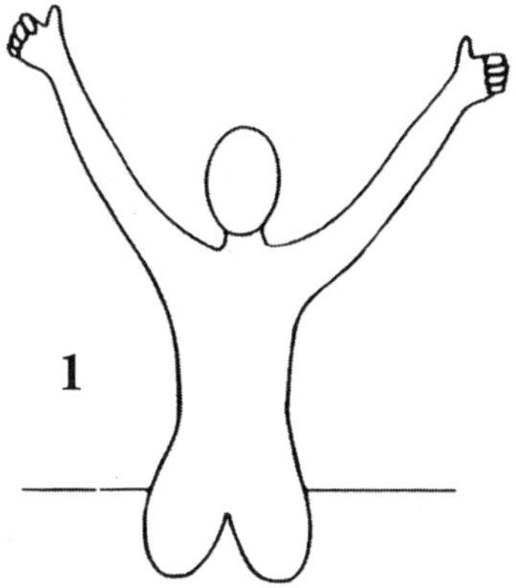

The following is not a set of yoga exercises. Each one is an individual technique that may be practiced on its own.

1. **Singh Praan Mudra** – Pose of Victory to the Four Corners of Infinity: Sit on your heels with your arms stretched out to the sides at a 60° angle. The four fingers are on the mounds and the thumb is sticking out. Make sure your elbows are straight. Keep your mouth open and stick out your tongue. Pump your navel without making any sound with your breath—not Breath of Fire. 3 Minutes.

To finish: Inhale and hold your breath for 10 seconds while you continue to pump your navel and stretch your arms out from your shoulders as far as possible. Repeat this two more times.

Do Singh Praan Mudra every day to build stamina and help you when you are tired and not at your best. It gives you the power to excel. Whoever shall master this meditation shall master the universe.

Yogi Bhajan

2

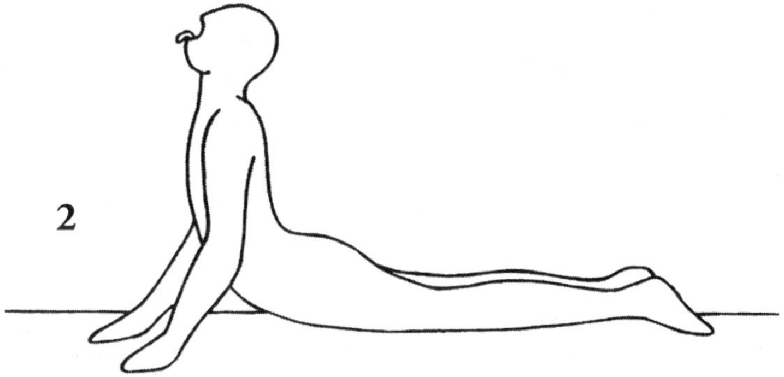

2. **To Get Out of Fatigue After Exertion:**
Get into Cobra Pose, stick out your tongue and do a rapid Breath of Fire for 1 minute only. Inhale deeply, hold your breath, come into a sitting position, stretch your hands upward, and release your breath.

3. **For Those Times When You Must Not Sleep:**
Train yourself to relax your mind and body so you can fall into deep sleep in Baby Pose for 5 Minutes. This conscious nap can enable you to work for 8 more hours.

3

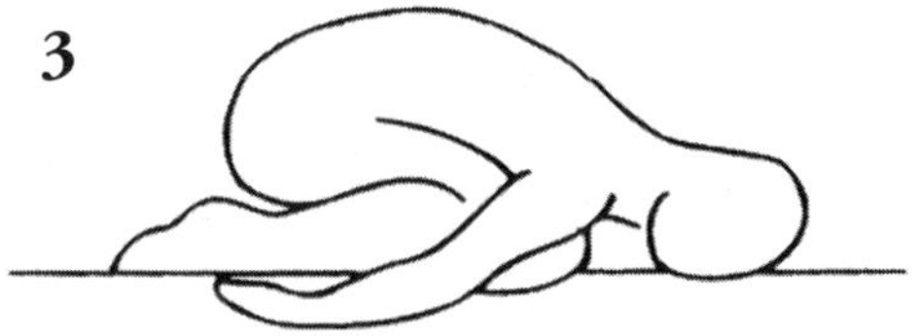

More Techniques to Fight Fatigue

July 1992

The following is not a set of yoga exercises. Each one is an individual technique that may be practiced on its own.

Never believe that the most neurotic, most ugly, most terrible situation is not testing you. It is testing your vastness, your wit, your capability, your flexibility your adjustment, and your character.

Yogi Bhajan

1. **To Stay Young:**
From a standing position, bend over and touch your wrists to your toes. Hold for 1-3 Minutes.

2. **To Renew Your Energy and Stimulate Circulation:**
Sit comfortably in Easy Pose: Do each exercise for 30 seconds to 1 minute

a. With open hands, rapidly hit the sides of your head.
b. With open hands, rapidly hit the back of your head.
c. With open hands, rapidly hit your thighs.
d. With both hands at the same time, rub your cheeks in a circular motion.
e. With one hand on your forehead and one hand on your chin, massage in a circular motion.
f. Massage all around your neck.

3. **Long Cross-Short Cross to Remove Fatigue After Walking and Marching Long Distances:**
Long Cross: Sitting with the legs stretched out in front with the ankles crossed.
Short Cross: Sitting in Easy Pose.
Begin by sitting in Long Cross, then pull your legs into short cross. Next lie back so your back is on the ground and your legs are still in Short Cross. Sit up in Short Cross, stand up without using your hands, and then sit down again in Short Cross. Repeat the whole sequence again beginning with Long Cross.

4. **Exercise Set to Relieve Fatigue After Exertion:**

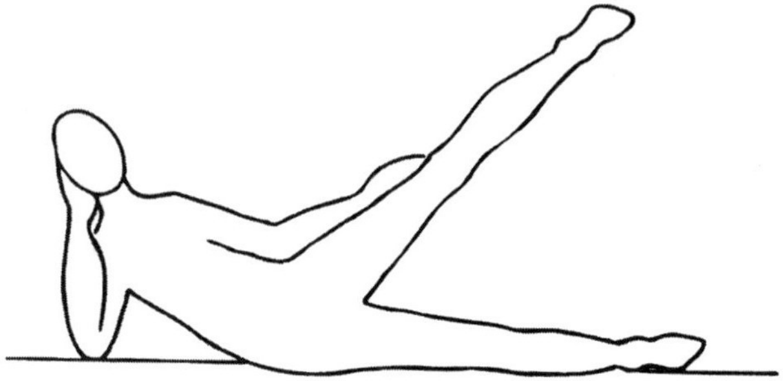

4a

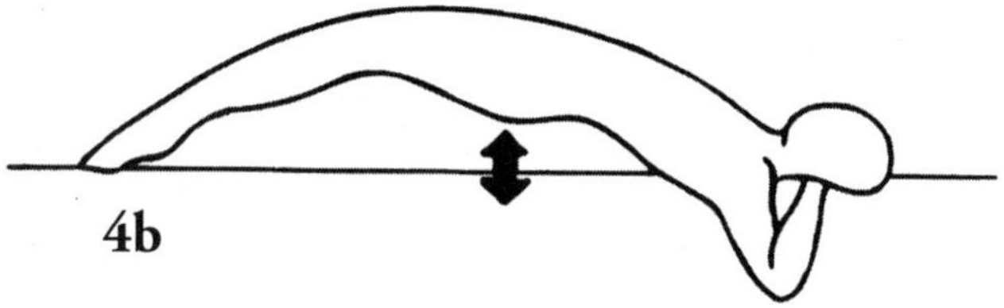

4b

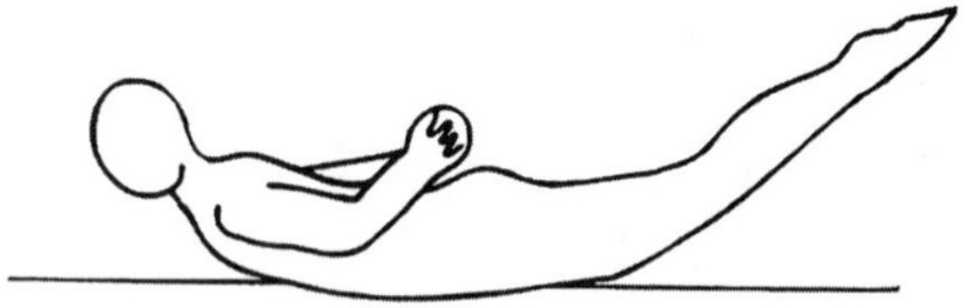

4c

a. Lie on your right side with your right hand supporting your head. Put your left arm on your left leg and raise your left leg up to 60°. Hold 1-3 Minutes.
b. Lie on your back with your hands under your head and rapidly jump your buttocks up and down. 1-3 Minutes.
c. Lie on your stomach with your fingers interlaced at the small of your back. Lift your head and legs and rock back and forth on your stomach. 1-3 Minutes.

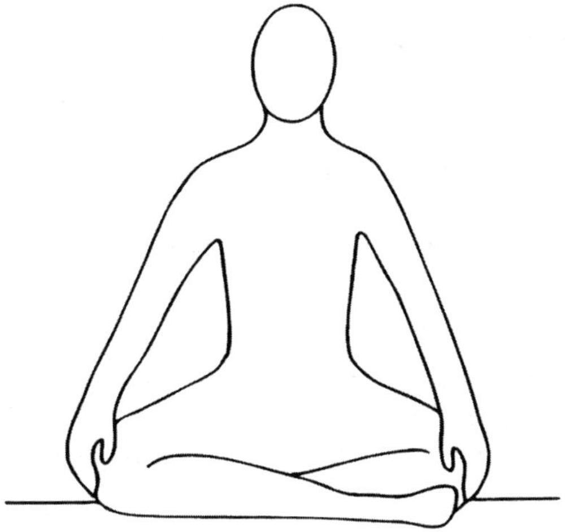

Ten Steps to Peace:

Remove Bad Memories and Painful Experiences

1. Lower the eyelids until the eyes are only open 1/10th. Concentrate on the tip of the nose. Silently say Wahe Guru in the following manner:
   Wha: mentally focus on the right eye. Hey: mentally focus on the left eye.
   Guru: mentally focus on the tip of the nose.
2. Inhale and remember the encounter or incident which happened to you.
3. Exhale and mentally say Wahe Guru in the above manner.
4. Inhale. Visualize and re-live the actual feeling of the encounter.
5. Exhale and again mentally repeat Wahe Guru.
6. Inhale and reverse roles in the encounter you are remembering. Become the other person and experience their perspective.
7. Exhale and mentally repeat Wahe Guru.
8. Inhale. Forgive the other person and forgive yourself.
9. Exhale and mentally repeat Wahe Guru.
10. Inhale. Let go of the incident and release it into the Universe.

This meditation takes care of phobias, fears, and neuroses. It can remove unsettling thoughts from the past that surface into the present. It can take difficult situations in the present and release them into the hands of Infinity. All this can be done in just forty seconds!

Yogi Bhajan

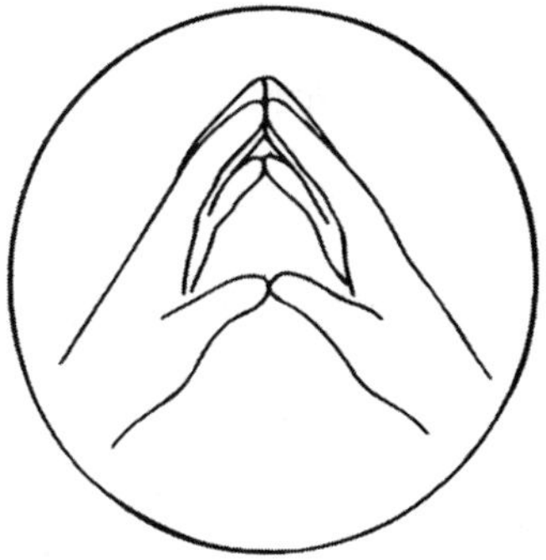

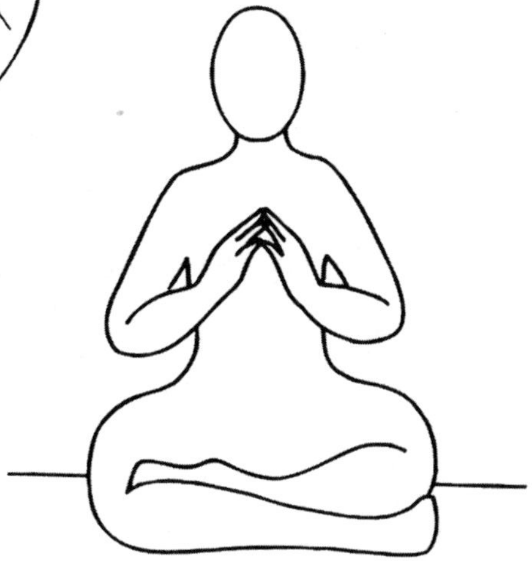

Stress Relief and Clearing the Emotions of the Past

Put your hands in front of your chest with the tips of the thumbs touching each other and each of the fingers touching the corresponding fingers on the opposite hand. There is space between the palms. The fingertips are pointing upward. Look at the tip of your nose and breathe 4 times per minute: inhale 5 seconds, hold 5 seconds, exhale 5 seconds. Continue for 11 Minutes or until you feel relief from the stress.

This meditation is especially useful for dealing with stressful relationships and with past family issues.

Appendix A

Music Used in the Yoga Sets

Ang Sang Wahe Guru by Nirinjan Kaur

Aquarian Sadhana by Wahe Guru Kaur

Bhor Na Marne Hoaa by Ragi Sat Nam Singh

Ek Ong Kar Sat Gur Prasad by Nirinjan Kaur

Guru Ram Das Lullaby

Har Har Har Har Gobinde by Nirinjan Kaur

Har Har Mukande with Affirmations by Liv Singh

Har Nar Wahe Guru by Nirinjan Kaur

Har Singh Nar Singh, Neel Narayan. by Nirinjan Kaur

Hummee Hum, Brahm Hum by Nirinjan Kaur

Jaap Sahib by Ragi Sat Nam Singh

Jai Te Gang by Bhai Avtar Singh and Bhai Gurucharan Singh

Last Four lines of Jaap Sahib (Chattr Chakkr Varti) by Nirinjan Kaur

Naad, the Blessing by Sangeet Kaur

Ong Namo Guru Dev Namo by Nirinjan Kaur

Rakhe Rakhanhar by Nirinjan Kaur

Sat Nam Wahe Guru (Indian version)

Walking up the Mountain by Gurudass Singh and Krishna Kaur

Music can be purchased from your local yoga center or the following mail order companies:

Music and Yogi Bhajan Lectures
Ancient Healing Ways
39 Shady Lane
Espanola, New Mexico 87532
877-853-5351
Store.a-healing.com

Music and books:
Spirit Voyage
www.spiritvoyage.com
888-735-4800

Resources

This and other KRI products are available from the Kundalini Research Institute (KRI):

www.kriteachings.org

Remember to always buy from 'The Source'!

For information regarding international events:

www.3HO.org

To find a teacher in your area or for more information about becoming a Kundalini Yoga teacher:

www.kundaliniyoga.com

Of further interest:

www.sikhnet.org

Kundalini Yoga as taught by Yogi Bhajan®

Kundalini Research Institute